Alan Brown (handwritten)

Handbook of Drugs in Intensive Care

A thoroughly updated edition of this well-established guide to drugs and prescribing for intensive care. The book is split into two sections: an A–Z guide to the drugs available, and concise notes on the key topics and situations faced on a daily basis. The A–Z section provides succinct information on each drug including uses, limitations, administration directions and adverse effects. The second section details complications that may arise in patients with particular conditions such as diabetes, epilepsy and renal failure, and other factors that may affect drug prescribing. There is also a section of key data, showing weight conversions, body mass index and corresponding dosage calculations. This edition includes a colour fold-out chart showing drug compatibility for intravenous administration. Presented in a concise, compact format, this book is an invaluable resource for doctors, nurses and other medical professionals caring for critically ill patients.

HENRY PAW is a consultant in anaesthesia and intensive care at York Hospital, York.

GILBERT PARK is a consultant in anaesthesia and intensive care at Addenbrooke's Hospital, Cambridge.

Paw ~ 40 (handwritten)

D0309713

Who's Book is this? Mine!! (handwritten)

Each O₂ litre gi' equivelant to approx 3% (handwritten)

This book is dedicated to Georgina Paw

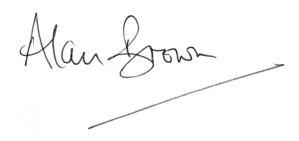

Handbook of
Drugs in Intensive Care:
An A-Z Guide

3rd ed

Henry G W Paw

BPharm MRPharmS MBBS FRCA
Consultant in Anaesthesia and Intensive Care
York Hospital
York

Gilbert R Park

MD DMedSci FRCA
Consultant in Anaesthesia and Intensive Care
Addenbrooke's Hospital
Cambridge

No Really who's Book is
this?

Pam s Now!

its not its
BROONIES!!!

Dave!!

Is this my book?

CAMBRIDGE UNIVERSITY PRESS
Cambridge, New York, Melbourne, Madrid, Cape Town, Singapore, São Paulo, Delhi

Cambridge University Press
The Edinburgh Building, Cambridge CB2 8RU, UK

Published in the United States of America by Cambridge University Press, New York

www.cambridge.org
Information on this title: www.cambridge.org/9780521687812

First published 2000
Reprinted 2001
Second Edition 2002
Third Edition 2006
Third printing 2008

Printed in the United Kingdom at the University Press, Cambridge

A catalogue record for this publication is available from the British Library

Library of Congress Cataloguing in Publication data

ISBN 978-0-521-68781-2 paperback

Mix antibiotics with WFI ✶

CONTENTS

INTRODUCTION

The main challenge when I embarked in writing the third edition has been to keep it down to size. This third edition remains a concise book that explains how to use drugs safely and effectively in a critical care setting. Doctors, nurses and other professionals caring for the critically ill patient will find it useful. It is intended to be small enough to fit in the pocket and to provide sufficient information about drug prescribing in the critically ill patient. To keep the book down to size has meant restricting the list of drugs to ones that I consider as common drugs. It is not intended to list every conceivable complication and problem that can occur with a drug but to concentrate on those the clinician is likely to encounter. These constraints mean that this pocket book should be seen as complementary to, rather than replacing, the standard textbooks.

The book is composed of two main sections. The A–Z guide is the major part and is arranged alphabetically by the non-proprietary name of the drug. This format has made it easier for the user to find a particular drug when in a hurry. The discussion on an individual drug is restricted to its use in the critically ill adult patient. The second part is comprised of short notes on relevant intensive care topics.

While every effort has been made to check drug dosages based on a 70 kg adult and information about every drug, it is still possible that errors may have crept in. I would therefore ask readers to check the information if it seems incorrect. In addition, I would be pleased to hear from any readers with suggestions about how this book can be improved. Comments should be sent via e-mail to: henry.paw@york.nhs.uk.

HGWP
York 2006

HOW TO USE THIS BOOK

European law (directive 92/27/EEC) requires the use of the Recommended International Non-proprietary Name (rINN) in place of the British Approved Name (BAN). For a small number of drugs these names are different. The Department of Health requires the use of BAN to cease and be replaced by rINN with the exceptions of adrenaline and noradrenaline. For these two drugs both their BAN and rINN will continue to be used.

The format of this book was chosen to make it more 'user friendly' – allowing the information to be readily available to the reader in times of need. For each drug there is a brief introduction, followed by the following categories:

Uses
This is the indication for the drug's use in the critically ill. There will be some unlicensed use included and this will be indicated in brackets.

Contraindications
This includes conditions or circumstances in which the drug should not be used – the contraindications. For every drug, this includes known hypersensitivity to the particular drug or its constituents.

Administration
This includes the route and dosage for a 70 kg adult. For obese patients, estimated ideal body weight should be used in the calculation of the dosage (Appendix D). It also advises on dilutions and situations where dosage may have to be modified. To make up a dilution, the instruction 'made up to 50 ml with 0.9% saline' means that the final volume is 50 ml. In contrast, the instruction 'to dilute with 50 ml 0.9% saline' could result in a total volume >50 ml. It is recommended that no drug should be stored for >24 h after reconstitution or dilution.

How not to use . . .
Describes administration techniques or solutions for dilution which are not recommended.

Adverse effects
These are effects other than those desired.

Cautions
Warns of situations when the use of the drug is not contraindicated but needs to be carefully watched. This will include drug-drug interactions.

Organ failure

Highlights any specific problems that may occur when using the drug in a particular organ failure.

Renal replacement therapy

Provides guidance on the effects of haemofiltration/dialysis on the handling of the drug. For some drugs, data are either limited or not available.

ABBREVIATIONS

ACE-I	angiotensin converting enzyme inhibitor
ACh	acetylcholine
ACT	activated clotting time
ADH	antidiuretic hormone
AF	atrial fibrillation
APTT	activated partial thromboplastin time
ARDS	acute respiratory distress syndrome
AV	atrioventricular
BP	blood pressure
CABG	coronary artery bypass graft
cAMP	cyclic AMP
CC	creatinine clearance
CMV	cytomegalovirus
CNS	central nervous system
CO	cardiac output
COPD	chronic obstructive pulmonary disease
CPR	cardiopulmonary resuscitation
CSF	cerebrospinal fluid
CT	computerised tomography
CVVH	continuous veno-venous haemofiltration
CVVHD	continuous veno-venous haemodiafiltration
DI	diabetes insipidus
DIC	disseminated intravascular coagulation
DVT	deep vein thrombosis
EBV	Epstein Barr virus
ECG	electrocardiogram
EEG	electroencephalogram
EMD	electromechanical dissociation
$ETCO_2$	end-tidal carbon dioxide concentration
FBC	full blood count
FFP	fresh frozen plasma
g	gram
GFR	glomerular filtration rate
GI	gastrointestinal
HOCM	hypertrophic obstructive cardiomyopathy
h	hour
HR	heart rate
ICP	intracranial pressure
ICU	intensive care unit
IHD	ischaemic heart disease
IM	intramuscular
INR	international normalised ratio
IOP	intraocular pressure
IPPV	intermittent positive pressure ventilation
IV	intravenous
K^+	potassium
kg	kilogram

l	litre
LFT	liver function tests
LMWH	low molecular weight heparin
MAOI	monoamine oxidase inhibitor
M6G	morphine-6-glucuronide
mg	milligram
MH	malignant hyperthermia
MI	myocardial infarction
MIC	minimum inhibitory concentration
min	minute
ml	millilitre
MRSA	methicillin-resistant *Staphylococcus aureus*
NG	nasogastric route
ng	nanogram
NJ	nasojejunal
nocte	at night
NSAID	non-steroidal anti-inflammatory drugs
PaO_2	partial pressure of oxygen in arterial blood
$PaCO_2$	partial pressure of carbon dioxide in arterial blood
PCAS	patient controlled analgesia system
PCP	*Pneumocystis carinii* pneumonia
PCWP	pulmonary capillary wedge pressure
PD	peritoneal dialysis
PE	pulmonary embolism
PEA	pulseless electrical activity
PEG	percutaneous endoscopic gastrostomy
PEJ	percutaneous endoscopic jejunostomy
PO	*per orum* (by mouth)
PR	*per rectum* (rectal route)
PRN	*pro re nata* (as required)
PVC	polyvinyl chloride
PVD	peripheral vascular disease
s	second
SC	subcutaneous
SIRS	systemic inflammatory response syndrome
SL	sublingual
SSRI	selective serotonin re-uptake inhibitors
SVR	systemic vascular resistance
SVT	supraventricular tachycardia
TFT	thyroid function tests
TNF	tumour necrosis factor
TPN	total parenteral nutrition
U&E	urea and electrolytes
VF	ventricular fibrillation
VRE	Vancomycin-resistant *Enterococcus faecium*
VT	ventricular tachycardia
WFI	water for injection
WPW syndrome	Wolff-Parkinson-White syndrome

ACKNOWLEDGEMENTS

I would like to thank all my colleagues from whom I have sought advice during the preparation of this book. In particular, I acknowledge the assistance of Dr Neil Todd for microbiological advice.

Drugs:
An A–Z Guide

Hypo**K**alaemia - the presence of abnormally
low levels of potassium
in the blood, occurs in
dehydration

Hypo**na**traemia - the presence in the
blood of an abnormally
low concentration of sodium,
occurs in dehydration

ACETAZOLAMIDE

Acetazolamide is a carbonic anhydrase inhibitor normally used to reduce intra-ocular pressure in glaucoma. Metabolic alkalosis may be partially corrected by the use of acetazolamide. The most common cause of metabolic alkalosis on the ICU is usually the result of furosemide administration.

Uses
Metabolic alkalosis (unlicensed)

Contraindications
Hypokalaemia
Hyponatraemia
Hyperchloraemic acidosis
Severe liver failure
Renal failure
Sulphonamide hypersensitivity

Administration
• IV: 250–500 mg, given over 3–5 min every 8 hours

Reconstitute with 5 ml WFI
Monitor: FBC, U&E and acid/base balance

How not to use acetazolamide
IM injection – painful
Not for prolonged use

Adverse effects
Metabolic acidosis
Electrolyte disturbances (hypokalaemia and hyponatraemia)
Blood disorders
Abnormal LFT

Cautions
Avoid extravasation at injection site (risk of necrosis)
Avoid prolonged use (risk of adverse effects)
Concurrent use with phenytoin (↑ serum level of phenytoin)

Organ failure
Renal: avoid (metabolic acidosis)
Hepatic: avoid (abnormal LFT)

ACETYLCYSTEINE (Parvolex)

Acetylcysteine is an effective antidote to paracetamol if administered within 8 h after an overdose. Although the protective effect diminishes progressively as the overdose – treatment interval increases, acetylcysteine can still be of benefit up to 24 h after the overdose. In paracetamol overdose the hepatotoxicity is due to formation of a toxic metabolite. Hepatic reduced glutathione inactivates the toxic metabolite by conjugation, but glutathione stores are depleted with hepatotoxic doses of paracetamol. Acetylcysteine, being a sulphydryl (SH) group donor, protects the liver probably by restoring depleted hepatic reduced glutathione or by acting as an alternative substrate for the toxic metabolite.

Acetylcysteine may have significant cytoprotective effects. The cellular damage associated with sepsis, trauma, burns, pancreatitis, hepatic failure and tissue reperfusion following acute MI may be mediated by the formation and release of large quantities of free radicals that overwhelm and deplete endogenous antioxidants (e.g. glutathione). Acetylcysteine is a scavenger of oxygen free radicals. In addition, acetylcysteine is a glutathione precursor capable of replenishing depleted intracellular glutathione and in theory augment antioxidant defences (p. 222).

Nebulized acetylcysteine can be used as a mucolytic agent. It reduces sputum viscosity by disrupting the disulphide bonds in the mucus glycoproteins and enhances mucociliary clearance, thus facilitating easier expectoration.

Uses
Paracetamol overdose
Antioxidant (unlicensed)
Reduce sputum viscosity and facilitate easier expectoration (unlicensed)
As a sulphydryl group donor to prevent the development of nitrate tolerance (unlicensed)

Administration

Paracetamol overdose

- IV infusion: 150 mg/kg in 200 ml 5% dextrose over 15 min, followed by 50 mg/kg in 500 ml 5% dextrose over 4 h, then 100 mg/kg in 1 litre 5% dextrose over the next 16 h

Weight (kg)	Initial	Second	Third
	150 mg/kg in 200 ml 5% dextrose over 15 min	50 mg/kg in 500 ml 5% dextrose over 4 h	100 mg/kg in 1 litre 5% dextrose over 16 h
	Parvolex (ml)	Parvolex (ml)	Parvolex (ml)
50	37.5	12.5	25
60	45.0	15.0	30
70	52.5	17.5	35
80	60.0	20.0	40
90	67.5	22.5	45
x	0.75x	0.25x	0.5x

For children >20 kg: same doses and regimen but in half the quantity of IV fluid

ACETYLCYSTEINE (Parvolex)

Treatment nomogram

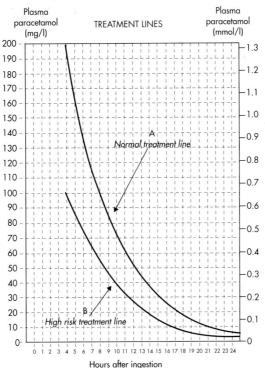

Patients whose plasma concentrations fall on or above treatment line A should receive acetylcysteine. Patients with induced hepatic microsomal oxidase enzymes (for chronic alcoholics and patients taking enzyme-inducing drugs, see p. 191) are susceptible to paracetamol-induced hepatotoxicity at lower paracetamol concentrations and should be assessed against treatment line B.

Antioxidant

• IV infusion: 75–100 mg/kg in 1 litre 5% dextrose, give over 24 h (rate 40 ml/h)

Reduce sputum viscosity

• Nebulized: 4 ml 800 mg undiluted Parvolex (20%) driven by air, 8 hourly

Administer before chest physiotherapy

How not to use acetylcysteine
Do not drive nebulizer with oxygen (oxygen inactivates acetylcysteine)

Adverse effects
Anaphylactoid reactions (nausea, vomiting, flushing, itching, rashes, bronchospasm, hypotension)
Fluid overload

Cautions
Asthmatics (risk of bronchospasm)
Pulmonary oedema (worsens)
Each 10 ml ampoule contains Na^+ 12.78 mmol ($\uparrow$ total body sodium)

ACICLOVIR (Zovirax)

Interferes with herpes virus DNA polymerase, inhibiting viral DNA replication. Aciclovir is renally excreted and has a prolonged half-life in renal impairment.

Uses

Herpes simplex virus infections:

HSV - Herpes Simplex Virus

- HSV encephalitis
- HSV genital, labial, peri-anal and rectal infections

Varicella zoster virus infections:

- Beneficial in the immunocompromised patients when given IV within 72 h: prevents complications of pneumonitis, hepatitis or thrombocytopenia
- In patients with normal immunity, may be considered if the ophthalmic branch of the trigeminal nerve is involved

Contraindications

Not suitable for CMV or EBV infections

Administration

- IV: 5–10 mg/kg 8 hourly

Available in 250 and 500 mg vials for reconstitution
Reconstitute 250 mg vial with 10 ml WFI or 0.9% saline (25 mg/ml)
Reconstitute 500 mg vial with 20 ml WFI or 0.9% saline (25 mg/ml)
Take the reconstituted solution (25 mg/ml) and make up to 50 ml (for 250 mg vial) or 100 ml (for 500 mg vial) with 0.9% saline or 5% dextrose, and give over 1 h
Ensure patient is well hydrated before treatment is administered
In renal impairment:

CC (ml/min)	Dose (mg/kg)	Interval (h)
10–20	5	12
<10	2.5	24

How not to use aciclovir

- Rapid IV infusion (precipitation of drug in renal tubules leading to renal impairment)

Adverse effects

Phlebitis
Reversible renal failure
Elevated liver function tests
CNS toxicity (tremors, confusion and fits)

Viral
treatment A

Cautions
Concurrent use of methotrexate
Renal impairment (reduce dose)
Dehydration/hypovolaemia (renal impairment due to precipitation in renal tubules)

Renal replacement therapy
Removed by HD and HF, similar to urea clearance. Elimination will only be significant for high clearance systems. Dose as for CC 10–25 ml/min. Not significantly cleared by PD.

Encephalitis – inflammation of the brain.

It may be caused by a viral or bacterial infection or it may be part of an allergic response to a systemic viral illness or vaccination

Thrombocytopenia – (TCP) a reduction in the number of platelets in the blood. This results in bleeding into the skin, spontaneous bruising & prolonged bleeding after injury

ACICLOVIR (ZOVIRAX)

g. for arrhythmia

ADENOSINE (Adenocor)

This endogenous nucleoside is safe and effective in ending >90% of re-entrant paroxysmal SVT. However, this is not the most common type of SVT in the critically ill patient. After an IV bolus effects are immediate (10–30 s), dose-related and transient (half-life <10 s; entirely eliminated from plasma in <1 min, being degraded by vascular endothelium and erythrocytes). Its elimination is not affected by renal/hepatic disease. Adenosine works faster and is superior to verapamil. It may be used in cardiac failure, in hypotension, and with β-blockers, in all of which verapamil is contraindicated.

Uses

It has both therapeutic and diagnostic uses:

- Alternative to DC cardioversion in terminating paroxysmal SVT, including those associated with WPW syndrome
- Determining the origin of broad complex tachycardia; SVT responds, VT does not (predictive accuracy 92%; partly because VT may occasionally respond). Though adenosine does no harm in VT, verapamil may produce hypotension or cardiac arrest

Contraindications

Second- or third-degree heart block (unless pacemaker fitted)
Sick sinus syndrome (unless pacemaker fitted)
Asthmatic – may cause bronchospasm
Patients on dipyridamole (drastically prolongs the half-life and enhances the effects of adenosine – may lead to dangerously prolonged high-degree AV block)

Administration

- Rapid IV bolus: 3 mg over 1–2 s into a large vein, followed by rapid flushing with 0.9% saline

If no effect within 2 min, give 6 mg
If no effect within 2 min, give 12 mg
If no effect, abandon adenosine
Need continuous ECG monitoring
More effective given via a central vein or into right atrium

How not to use adenosine

Without continuous ECG monitor

Adverse effects

Flushing (18%), dyspnoea (12%), and chest discomfort are the commonest side-effects but are well tolerated and invariably last <1 min. If given to an asthmatic and bronchospasm occurs, this may last up to 30 min (use aminophylline to reverse).

A

Cautions

AF or atrial flutter with accessory pathway (↑ conduction down anomalous pathway may increase)

Early relapse of paroxysmal SVT is more common than with verapamil but usually responds to further doses

Adenosine's effect is enhanced and extended by dipyridamole − if essential to give with dipyridamole, reduce initial dose to 0.5−1.0 mg

Rapid reversion to sinus rhythm of paroxysmal supraventricular tachycardias, including those associated with accessory conducting pathways (eg. Wolff-Parkinson-White Syndrome); aid to diagnosis of broad or narrow complex supraventricular tachycardias

SVT- supraventricular tachycardia

ADRENALINE (Epinephrine).

Both α- and β-adrenergic receptors are stimulated. Low doses tend to produce predominantly β-effects while higher doses tend to produce predominantly α-effects. Stimulation of β_1-receptors in the heart increases the rate and force of contraction, resulting in an increase in cardiac output. Stimulation of α_1-receptor causes peripheral vasoconstriction, which increases the systolic BP. Stimulation of β_2-receptors causes bronchodilatation and vasodilatation in certain vascular beds (skeletal muscles). Consequently, total systemic resistance may actually fall, explaining the decrease in diastolic BP that is sometimes seen.

Uses
Low cardiac output states
Cardiac arrest (p. 198)
Anaphylaxis (p. 200)

Contraindications
Before adequate intravascular volume replacement

Administration
Low cardiac output states
Dose: 0.01–0.30 mcg/kg/min IV infusion via a central vein
Titrate dose according to HR, BP, cardiac output, presence of ectopic beats and urine output
4 mg made up to 50 ml 5% dextrose

Dosage chart (ml/h)

Weight (kg)	Dose (mcg/kg/min)				
	0.02	0.05	0.1	0.15	0.2
50	0.8	1.9	3.8	5.6	7.5
60	0.9	2.3	4.5	6.8	9.0
70	1.1	2.6	5.3	7.9	10.5
80	1.2	3.0	6.0	9.0	12
90	1.4	3.4	6.8	10.1	13.5
100	1.5	3.8	7.5	11.3	15.0
110	1.7	4.1	8.3	12.4	16.5
120	1.8	4.5	9.0	13.5	18.0

Cardiac arrest (p. 198)
- IV bolus: 10 ml 1 in 10 000 solution (1 mg).

ADRENALINE

Anaphylaxis (p. 200)

- IV bolus: 0.5–1.0 ml 1 in 10 000 solution (50–100 mcg), may be repeated PRN, according to BP

How not to use adrenaline
In the absence of haemodynamic monitoring
Do not connect to CVP lumen used for monitoring pressure (surge of drug during flushing of line)
Incompatible with alkaline solutions, e.g. sodium bicarbonate, frusemide, phenytoin and enoximone

Adverse effects
Arrhythmia
Tachycardia
Hypertension
Myocardial ischaemia

Cautions
Acute myocardial ischaemia or MI

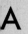

ALFENTANIL

It is 30 times more potent than morphine and its duration is shorter than that of fentanyl. The maximum effect occurs about 1 min after IV injection. Duration of action following an IV bolus is between 5 and 10 min. Its distribution volume and lipophilicity are lower than fentanyl. It is ideal for infusion and may be the agent of choice in renal failure. The context sensitive half-life may be prolonged following IV infusion. In patients with hepatic failure the elimination half-life may be markedly increased and a prolonged duration of action may be seen.

Uses
Patients receiving short-term ventilation

Contraindications
Airway obstruction
Concomitant use of MAOI

Administration
- IV bolus: 500 mcg every 10 min as necessary
- IV infusion rate: 1–5 mg/h (up to 1 mcg/kg/min)

How not to use alfentanil
In combination with an opioid partial agonist, e.g. buprenorphine (antagonizes opioid effects)

Adverse effects
Respiratory depression and apnoea
Bradycardia
Nausea and vomiting
Delayed gastric emptying
Reduce intestinal mobility
Biliary spasm
Constipation
Urinary retention
Chest wall rigidity (may interfere with ventilation)

Usually 25mg made up with 20 ml Nacl TV. 25mls

Cautions

Enhanced sedative and respiratory depression from interaction with:

- benzodiazepines
- antidepressants
- anti–psychotics

Avoid concomitant use of and for 2 weeks after MAOI discontinued (risk of CNS excitation or depression – hypertension, hyperpyrexia, convulsions and coma)

Head injury and neurosurgical patients (may exacerbate ↑ ICP as a result of ↑ $PaCO_2$)
Erythromycin (↓ clearance of alfentanil)

Organ failure

Respiratory: ↑ respiratory depression
Hepatic: enhanced and prolonged sedative effect

Analgesia especially during short operative procedure & outpatient surgery; enhancement of anaesthesia; analgesia & suppression of respiratory activity in pts receiving intensive care with assisted ventilation

A

ALFENTANIL

ALTEPLASE

The use of thrombolytics is well established in myocardial infarction. They act by activating plasminogen to form plasmin, which degrades fibrin and so breaks up thrombi. Alteplase or tissue-type plasminogen activator (rt-PA) can be used in major pulmonary embolism associated with hypoxia and haemodynamic compromise. Whilst alteplase is more expensive than streptokinase, it is the preferred thrombolytic as it does not worsen hypotension. Severe bleeding is a potential adverse effect of alteplase and requires discontinuation of the thrombolytic and may require administration of coagulation factors and antifibrinolytic drugs (aprotinin and tranexamic acid).

Uses
Major pulmonary embolism

Contraindications
Recent haemorrhage, trauma, or surgery
Coagulation defects
Severe hypertension
Oesophageal varices
Severe liver disease
Acute pancreatitis

Administration
• Pulmonary embolism

IV: 10 mg, given over 1–2 min, followed by IV infusion of 90 mg over 2 hours
Dissolve in WFI to a concentration of 1 mg/ml (50 mg vial with 50 ml WFI)
Monitor: BP (treat if systolic BP > 180 mmHg or diastolic BP > 105 mmHg)

How not to use alteplase
Not to be infused in glucose solution

Adverse effects
Nausea and vomiting
Bleeding

Cautions
Acute stroke (risk of cerebral bleed)
Diabetic retinopathy (risk of retinal bleeding)
Abdominal aortic aneurysm and enlarged left atrium with AF (risk of embolisation)

Organ failure
Renal: risk of hyperkalaemia
Hepatic: avoid in severe liver failure

AMINOPHYLLINE

The ethylenediamine salt of theophylline. It is a non-specific inhibitor of phosphodiesterase, producing increased levels of cAMP. Increased cAMP levels result in:

- Bronchodilation
- CNS stimulation
- Positive inotropic and chronotropic effects
- Diuresis

Theophylline has been claimed to reduce fatigue of diaphragmatic muscles

Uses
Prevention and treatment of bronchospasm

Contraindications
Uncontrolled arrhythmias
Hyperthyroidism

Administration
- Loading dose: 5 mg/kg IV, given over 30 min, followed by maintenance dose 0.1–0.8 mg/kg/h

Dilute 1 g (40 ml) aminophylline (25 mg/ml) in 460 ml 5% dextrose or 0.9% saline to give a concentration of 2 mg/ml
No loading dose if already on oral theophylline preparations (toxicity)
Reduce maintenance dose (0.1–0.3 mg/kg/h) in the elderly and patients with congestive heart failure and liver disease
Increase maintenance dose (0.8–1 mg/kg/h) in children (6 months – 16 years) and young adult smokers
Monitor plasma level (p. 193)
Therapeutic range 55–110 mmol/l or 10–20 mg/l

A

AMINOPHYLLINE

Dosage chart: ml/hr

Weight: Kg	Dose: mg/kg/hour									
	0.1	0.2	0.3	0.4	0.5	0.6	0.7	0.8	0.9	1
50	2.5	5	7.5	10	12.5	15	17.5	20	22.5	25
60	3	6	9	12	15	18	21	24	27	30
70	3.5	7	10.5	14	17.5	21	24.5	28	31.5	35
80	4	8	12	16	20	24	28	32	36	40
90	4.5	9	13.5	18	22.5	27	31.5	36	40.5	45
100	5	10	15	20	25	30	35	40	45	50
110	5.5	11	16.5	22	27.5	33	38.5	44	49.5	55
120	6	12	18	24	30	36	42	48	54	60
	• Elderly • Congestive Heart Failure • Liver disease			• Usual adult maintenance			• Children • Young adult smokers			

How not to use aminophylline
Rapid IV administration (hypotension, arrhythmias)

Adverse effects
Tachycardia
Arrhythmias
Convulsions

Cautions
Subject to enzyme inducers and inhibitors (p. 191)
Concurrent use of erythromycin and ciprofloxacin: reduce dose

Organ failure
Cardiac: prolonged half-life (reduce dose)
Hepatic: prolonged half-life (reduce dose)

AMIODARONE

Amiodarone has a broad-spectrum of activity on the heart. In addition to having an anti-arrhythmic activity, it also has anti-anginal effects. This may result from its α- and β-adrenoceptor blocking properties as well as from its calcium channel blocking effect in the coronary vessels. It causes minimal myocardial depression. It is therefore often a first-line drug in critical care situations. It has an extremely long half-life (15–105 days). Unlike oral amiodarone, IV administration usually acts relatively rapidly (20–30 min).

Uses
Good results with both ventricular and supraventricular arrhythmias, including those associated with WPW syndrome.

Contraindications
Iodine sensitivity (amiodarone contains iodine)
Sinus bradycardia (risk of asystole)
Heart block (unless pacemaker fitted)

Administration
- Loading: 300 mg in 250 ml 5% dextrose IV over 20–120 min, followed by 900 mg in .500 ml 5% dextrose over 24 h
- Maintenance: 600 mg IV daily for 7 days, then 400 mg IV daily for 7 days, then 200 mg IV daily

Administer IV via central line
Continuous cardiac monitoring

- Oral: 200 mg 8 hourly for 7 days, then 200 mg 12 hourly for 7 days, then 200 mg daily

How not to use amiodarone
Incompatible with 0.9% saline
Do not use peripheral vein (thrombophlebitis)

Adverse effects
Short-term
Skin reactions common
Vasodilation and hypotension or bradycardia after rapid infusion
Corneal microdeposits (reversible on stopping)
Long-term
Pulmonary fibrosis, alveolitis and pneumonitis (usually reversible on stopping)
Liver dysfunction (asymptomatic ↑ in LFT common)
Hypo- or hyperthyroidism (check TFT before starting drug)
Peripheral neuropathy, myopathy and cerebellar dysfunction (reversible on stopping)

Cautions
Increased risk of bradycardia, AV block and myocardial depression with
β-blockers and calcium-channel antagonists
Potentiates the effect of digoxin, theophylline and warfarin – reduce dose

Organ failure
Hepatic: worsens
Renal: accumulation of iodine may ↑ risk of thyroid dysfunction

AMITRIPTYLINE

A tricyclic antidepressant with sedative properties. When given at night it will help to promote sleep. It may take up to 2 weeks before any beneficial effect is seen unless a large loading dose is used.

Uses
Depression in patients requiring long-term ICU stay, particularly where sedation is required
Difficulty with sleep

Contraindications
Recent myocardial infarction
Arrhythmia
Heart block
Severe liver disease

Administration
- Oral: 25–75 mg nocte
- IM/IV bolus: 10–20 mg nocte

How not to use amitriptyline
During the daytime (disturbs the normal sleep pattern)

Adverse effects
Antimuscarinic effects (dry mouth, blurred vision, urinary retention)
Arrhythmias
Postural hypotension
Confusion
Hyponatraemia

Cautions
Cardiac disease (risk of arrhythmias)
Hepatic failure
Acute angle glaucoma
Concurrent use of MAOI
Additive CNS depression with other sedative agents
May potentiate direct-acting sympathomimetic drugs
Prostatic hypertrophy – urinary retention (unless patient's bladder catheterized)

Organ failure
CNS: sedative effects increased
Hepatic: sedative effects increased

AMPHOTERICIN (Fungizone)

Amphotericin is active against most fungi and yeasts. It is not absorbed from the gut when given orally. When given IV it is highly toxic and side-effects are common. The liposomal and colloidal formulations now available are less toxic, particularly in terms of nephrotoxicity.

Uses
Suppress gut carriage of Candida species by the oral route
Severe systemic fungal infections:
    Aspergillosis
    Candidiasis
    Coccidiomycosis
    Cryptococcosis
    Histoplasmosis

Administration
• Oral: suppression of gut carriage of Candida
100–200 mg 6 hourly

• IV: systemic fungal infections

Initial test dose of 1 mg given over 30 min, then 250 mcg/kg daily, gradually increased if tolerated to 1 mg/kg daily

• For severe infection: 1.5 mg/kg daily or on alternate days

Available in 20 ml vial containing 50 mg amphotericin
Reconstitute with 10 ml WFI (5 mg/ml), then further dilute the reconstituted solution as follows:

For peripheral administration:
    Dilute further with 500 ml 5% dextrose (to 0.1 mg/ml)
    Give over 6 h

For central administration:
    Dilute further with 50–100 ml 5% dextrose
    Give over 6 h

Prolonged treatment usually needed (duration depends on severity and nature of infection)

Monitor:
Serum potassium, magnesium and creatinine
FBC
LFT

How not to use amphotericin
Must not be given by rapid IV infusion (arrhythmias)
Not compatible with saline

A

Adverse effects
Fever and rigors – common in first week. May need paracetamol, chlorpheniramine and hydrocortisone premedication
Nephrotoxicity – major limiting toxicity. Usually reversible
Hypokalaemia/hypomagnesaemia – 25% will need supplements
Anaemia (normochromic, normocytic) – 75%. Due to bone marrow suppression
Cardiotoxicity – arrhythmias and hypotension with rapid IV bolus
Phlebitis – frequent change of injection site
Pulmonary reactions
GI upset – anorexia, nausea, vomiting

Cautions
Kidney disease
Concurrent use of other nephrotoxic drugs
Hypokalaemia – increased digoxin toxicity
Avoid concurrent administration of corticosteroids (except to treat febrile and anaphylactic reactions)

Organ failure
Renal: use only if no alternative; nephrotoxicity may be reduced with use of Amphocil or AmBisome

Renal replacement therapy
No further dose modification is required during renal replacement therapy

AMPHOTERICIN (Fungizone)

AMPHOTERICIN (COLLOIDAL) – Amphocil

Amphocil is a colloidal formulation containing a stable complex of amphotericin and sodium cholesteryl sulphate. It is available in vials containing either 50 or 100 mg amphotericin. This renders the drug less toxic to the kidney than the parent compound. Deterioration in renal function attributable to amphocil is rare.

Uses
Severe systemic fungal infections, when conventional amphotericin is contraindicated because of toxicity, especially nephrotoxicity.

Administration
- IV infusion: start at 1 mg/kg once daily, increasing to 3–4 mg/kg once daily, given over 60–90 min

Amphocil must be initially reconstituted by adding WFI:
    50 mg vial – add 10 ml WFI
    100 mg vial – add 20 ml WFI

The liquid in each reconstituted vial will contain 5 mg/ml amphotericin. This is further diluted to a final concentration of 0.625 mg/ml by diluting 1 volume of the reconstituted amphocil with 7 volumes 5% dextrose
Flush an existing intravenous line with 5% dextrose before infusion
Although anaphylactic reactions rare, before starting treatment, an initial test dose of 2 mg should be given over 10 min, infusion stopped and patient observed for 30 min. Continue infusion if no signs of anaphylactic reaction.
Monitor: Serum potassium and magnesium
In renal dialysis patients, give amphocil at the end of each dialysis

How not to use colloidal amphotericin
Must not be given by rapid IV infusion (arrhythmias)
Not compatible with saline
Do not mix with other drugs

Adverse effects
Prevalence and severity lower than conventional amphotericin

Cautions
Kidney disease
Concurrent use of nephrotoxic drugs
Avoid concurrent administration of corticosteroids (except to treat febrile and anaphylactic reactions)
Diabetes: amphocil contains lactose monohydrate 950 mg/50 mg vial or 1900 mg/100 mg vial (may cause hyperglycaemia)

AMPHOTERICIN (LIPOSOMAL) – AmBisome

A formulation of amphotericin encapsulated in liposomes. This renders the drug less toxic to the kidney than the parent compound. Each vial contains 50 mg amphotericin. Store vials in fridge between 2 and 8°C.

Uses
Severe systemic fungal infections, when conventional amphotericin is contraindicated because of toxicity, especially nephrotoxicity.

Administration
- IV: initially 1 mg/kg daily, ↑ gradually if necessary to 3 mg/kg daily

Add 12 ml WFI to each 50 mg vial of liposomal amphotericin (4 mg/ml) Shake vigorously for at least 15 s
Calculate the amount of the 4 mg/ml solution required, i.e.:
> 100 mg = 25 ml
> 150 mg = 37.5 ml
> 200 mg = 50 ml
> 300 mg = 75 ml

Using the 5 micron filter provided add the required volume of the 4 mg/ml solution to at least equal volume of 5% dextrose (final concentration 2 mg/ml) and given over 30–60 min
Although anaphylactic reactions rare, before starting treatment an initial test dose of 1 mg should be given over 10 min, infusion stopped and patient observed for 30 min. Continue infusion if no signs of anaphylactic reaction
The diluted solution must be used within 6 h
Monitor: Serum potassium and magnesium
In renal dialysis patients, give amBisome at the end of each dialysis

How not to use liposomal amphotericin
Must not be given by rapid IV infusion (arrhythmias)
Not compatible with saline
Do not mix with other drugs

Adverse effects
Prevalence and severity lower than conventional amphotericin

Cautions
Kidney disease
Concurrent use of nephrotoxic drugs
Avoid concurrent administration of corticosteroids (except to treat febrile and anaphylactic reactions)
Diabetic patient: each vial contains 900 mg sucrose

AMPICILLIN

Ampicillin has a spectrum of activity, which includes staphylococci, streptococci, most enterococci, *Listeria monocytogenes* and Gram −ve rods such as *Salmonella* spp., *Shigella* spp., *E. coli, H. influenzae and Proteus* spp. It is not active against *Pseudomnas aeruginosa and Klebsiella spp.* However due to acquired resistance almost all staphylococci, 50% of *E. coli* and up to 15% of *H. influenzae strains* are now resistant. Amoxicillin is similar but better absorbed orally.

Uses
Urinary tract infections
Respiratory tract infections
Invasive salmonellosis
Serious infections with *Listeria monocytogenes* including meningitis

Contraindications
Penicillin hypersensitivity

Administration
• IV: 0.5–1 g diluted in 10 ml WFI, 4–6 hourly over 3–5 min

In renal impairment:

CC (ml/min)	Dose (g)	Interval (hr)
10–20	0.5–1	8
<10	0.5–1	12

• Meningitis caused by *Listeria monocytogenes* (with gentamicin)

IV: 2 g diluted in 10 ml WFI every 4 hours over 3–5 min. Treat for 10–14 days

How not to use ampicillin
Not for intrathecal use (encephalopathy)
Do not mix in the same syringe with an aminoglycoside (efficacy of aminoglycoside reduced)

Adverse effects
Hypersensitivity
Skin rash increases in patients with infectious mononucleosis (90%), chronic lymphocytic leukaemia and HIV infections (discontinue drug)

Cautions
Severe renal impairment (reduce dose, rashes more common)

Renal replacement therapy
Removed by HD/HF/PD but significant only for high clearance technique. Dose as for CC 10–20 ml/min

APROTININ (Trasylol)

Aprotinin is a polypeptide derived from bovine lung. The mechanisms producing the decrease in blood loss are unclear but may be due to its inhibition of plasmin and preservation of platelet membrane-binding receptors. On the other hand there is no risk of developing DVT with its use, due to its weak anticoagulant effect. The current cost is £19 per 50 ml vial (500 000 units), compared with approximately £90 for one unit of blood.

Uses

Blood conservation – established role in open heart surgery and liver transplants. There are some promising reports of its use in orthopaedic procedures and in the critically ill
Uncontrolled bleeding caused by hyperplasminaemia

Contraindications

Known hypersensitivity

Administration

Blood conservation

- IV infusion: loading dose of 200 ml (2 million units) given over 30 min. The initial 5 ml (50 000 units) should be given slowly, over 5 min, due to the small risk of hypersensitivity reactions

If necessary, further 50 ml (500 000 units) every hour may be given
Uncontrolled bleeding due to hyperplasminaemia (not correctable by blood products)

- IV infusion: loading dose of 50 ml (500 000 units) to 100 ml (1 million units) given over 20 min. The initial 5 ml (50 000 units) should be given slowly, over 5 min, due to the small risk of hypersensitivity reactions

If necessary, further 20 ml (200 000 units) every hour may be given until bleeding stops

Adverse effects

Generally well tolerated
Thrombophlebitis
Hypersensitivity

Cautions

Incompatible with corticosteroids, heparin, nutrient solutions containing amino acids or fat emulsions, and tetracyclines

neuromuscular blockade for surgery or during Intensive Care

A

✱ ATRACURIUM

Atracurium is a non-depolarizing neuromuscular blocker that is broken down by Hofmann degradation and ester hydrolysis. The ampoules have to be stored in the fridge to prevent spontaneous degradation. Atracurium has an elimination half-life of 20 min. The principal metabolite is laudanosine, which can cause convulsions in dogs. Even with long-term infusions, the concentration of laudanosine is well below the seizure threshold (17 microgram/ml). It is the agent of choice in renal and hepatic failure.

Uses
Muscle paralysis

✱ *Standby when extubating*

Contraindications
Airway obstruction
✱ To facilitate tracheal intubation in patients at risk of regurgitation ✱

Administration
- IV bolus: 0.5 mg/kg, repeat with 0.15 mg/kg at 20–45 min interval
- IV infusion: 0.2–0.4 mg/kg/h

Monitor with peripheral nerve stimulator

How not to use atracurium
As part of a rapid sequence induction
In the conscious patient
By persons not trained to intubate trachea

Adverse effects
Bradycardia
Hypotension

Cautions
Asthmatics (histamine release)
Breathing circuit (disconnection)
Prolonged use (disuse muscle atrophy)

Organ failure
Hepatic: increased concentration of laudanosine
Renal: increased concentration of laudanosine

Given as a bolus !!

Reversal of excessive bradycardia

ATROPINE

The influence of atropine is most noticeable in healthy young adults in whom vagal tone is considerable. In infancy and old age, even large doses may fail to accelerate the heart.

Uses
Asystole (p. 198)
EMD or PEA with ventricular rate <60/min (p. 198)
Sinus bradycardia – will increase BP as a result
Reversal of muscarinic effects of anticholinesterases (neostigmine)
Organophosphate poisoning

Contraindications
Complete heart block
Tachycardia

Administration
- Bradycardia: 0.3–1 mg IV bolus, up to 3 mg (total vagolytic dose), may be diluted with WFI
- Asystole: 3 mg IV bolus, once only (p. 198)
- EMD or PEA with ventricular rate <60/min: 3 mg IV bolus, once only (p. 198)
- Reversal of muscarinic effects of anticholinesterase: 1.2 mg for every 2.5 mg neostigmine
- Organophosphate poisoning: 1–2 mg initially, then further 1–2 mg every 30 min PRN

How not to use atropine
Slow IV injection of doses <0.3 mg (bradycardia caused by medullary vagal stimulation)

Adverse effects
Drowsiness, confusion
Dry mouth
Blurred vision
Urinary retention
Tachycardia
Pyrexia (suppression of sweating)
Atrial arrhythmias and atrioventricular dissociation (without significant cardiovascular symptoms)
Dose >5 mg results in restlessness and excitation, hallucinations, delirium and coma

Cautions
Elderly (↑ CNS side-effects)
Child with pyrexia (further ↑ temperature)
Acute myocardial ischaemia or MI (tachycardia may cause worsening)
Prostatic hypertrophy – urinary retention (unless patient's bladder catheterized)
Paradoxically, bradycardia may occur at low doses (<0.3 mg)
Acute-angle glaucoma (further ↑ IOP)
Pregnancy (foetal tachycardia)

BENZYLPENICILLIN

Benzylpenicillin can only be given parenterally. It is active against most streptococci but the majority of strains of *Staphylococcus aureus* are resistant due to penicillinase production. Resistance rates are increasing in *Streptococcus pneumoniae* and benzylpenicillin should probably not be used for empiric treatment of meningitis unless local levels of resistance are extremely low. All strains of *Neisseria meningitidis* remain sensitive.

Uses
- Infective endocarditis
- Streptococcal infections including severe necrotising soft tissue infections and severe pharyngeal infections
- Pneumococcal infections – excluding empiric therapy of meningitis
- Gas gangrene and prophylaxis in limb amputation
- Meningococcal meningitis with sensitive organism
- Tetanus
- Prophylaxis post splenectomy

Contraindications
Penicillin hypersensitivity

Administration
IV: 600–1200 mg diluted in 10 ml WFI, 6 hourly over 3–5 min, higher doses should be given for severe infections
Give at a rate not >300 mg/min
Infective endocarditis: 7.2 g/24 h (with gentamicin)
Adult meningitis: 14.4 g/24 h

In renal impairment:

CC (ml/min)	Dose
10–20	75%
<10	20–50%

How not to use benzylpenicillin
Not for intrathecal use (encephalopathy)
Do not mix in the same syringe with an aminoglycoside (efficacy of aminoglycoside reduced)

B

Adverse effects
Hypersensitivity
Haemolytic anaemia
Transient neutropenia and thrombocytopenia
Convulsions (high-dose or renal failure)

Cautions
Anaphylactic reactions frequent (1:100 000)
Severe renal impairment (reduce dose, high-doses may cause convulsions)

Renal replacement therapy
Removed by HD/HF/PD but significant only for high clearance techniques
Dose as for CC 10–20 ml/min (75% dose)

BUMETANIDE

A loop diuretic similar to frusemide but 40 times more potent. Ototoxicity may be less with bumetanide than with frusemide, but nephrotoxicity may be worse.

Uses
- Acute oliguric renal failure
- May convert acute oliguric to non-oliguric renal failure. Other measures must be taken to ensure adequate circulating blood volume and renal perfusion pressure
- Pulmonary oedema secondary to acute left ventricular failure
- Oedema associated with congestive cardiac failure, hepatic failure and renal disease

Contraindications
Oliguria secondary to hypovolaemia

Administration
- IV bolus: 1–2 mg 1–2 min, repeat in 2–3 h if needed
- IV infusion: 2–5 mg in 100 ml 5% dextrose or 0.9% saline, given over 30–60 min

Adverse effects
Hyponatraemia, hypokalaemia, hypomagnesaemia
Hyperuricaemia, hyperglycaemia
Hypovolaemia
Ototoxicity
Nephrotoxicity
Pancreatitis

Cautions
Amphotericin (increased risk of hypokalaemia)
Aminoglycosides (increased nephrotoxicity and ototoxicity)
Digoxin toxicity (due to hypokalaemia)

Organ failure
Renal: may need to increase dose for effect

Renal replacement therapy
No further dose modification is required during renal replacement therapy

CAPTOPRIL

ACE inhibitors have a beneficial role in all grades of heart failure, combined when appropriate with diuretic and digoxin treatment.

Uses
Hypertension
Heart failure

Contraindications
Aortic stenosis
HOCM
Porphyria
Angioedema (idiopathic or hereditary)
Known or suspected renal artery stenosis (coexisting diabetes, PVD, hypertension)

Administration
- Orally: 6.25 mg trial, then 12.5–25 mg 8–12 hourly (maximum 50 mg 8 hourly)

Monitor:
> BP
> Serum potassium and creatinine

In mild to moderate renal impairment (CC 10–50 ml/min): 12.5 mg 12 hourly

Cautions
Risk of sudden and precipitous fall in BP in the following patients:
> Dehydrated
> Salt depleted (Na^+ <130 mmol/l)
> High dose diuretics (>80 mg frusemide daily)

Concomitant NSAID (↑ risk of renal damage)
Concomitant potassium-sparing diuretics (hyperkalaemia)
Peripheral vascular disease or generalized atherosclerosis (risk of clinically silent renovascular disease)

Adverse effects
Hypotension
Tachycardia
Dry cough
Rash
Pancreatitis
Altered LFT
Acidosis
Angioedema

Organ failure
Renal: reduce dose; hyperkalaemia more common

Renal replacement therapy
No further dose modification is required during renal replacement therapy

CASPOFUNGIN

Covers a wider range of Candida species causing invasive candidiasis than fluconazole and active against Aspergillus species. It has a better side effect profile than amphotericin. Side-effects are typically mild and rarely lead to discontinuation.

Uses
Invasive candidiasis
Invasive aspergillosis

Contraindications
Breast feeding

Administration
• IV: Load with 70 mg on day 1, followed by 50 mg daily thereafter for a minimum of 14 days

If >80 kg, continue with maintenance dose of 70 mg daily
If <70 kg, load with 50 mg, followed by 50 mg daily thereafter

Reconstitute with 10 ml WFI. Add the reconstituted solution to a 100 ml or 250 ml bag of 0.9% saline or Hartmann's solution, given over 1 hour.

Available in vials containing 50 mg and 70 mg powder. Store vials in fridge at 2–8°C.

How not to use caspofungin
Do not use diluents containing glucose

Adverse effects
Thrombophlebitis
Fever
Headache
Tachycardia
Anaemia
Decreased platelet count
Elevated LFT
Hypokalaemia
Hypomagnesaemia

Organ failure
Renal: No dose adjustment necessary
Hepatic: Mild (Child-Pugh score 5–6): No dose adjustment
       Moderate (Child-Pugh score 7–9): 70 mg loading followed by 35 mg daily
       Severe (Child-Pugh score >9): No data

Organ replacement therapy
Not removed by dialysis

CEFOTAXIME

A third generation cephalosporin with enhanced activity against Gram −ve species in comparison to second generation cephalosporins. It is not active against *Pseudomonas aeruginosa*, enterococci or *Bacteroides* spp. Use is increasingly being compromised by the emergence of Gram −ve strains expressing extended spectrum beta-lactamases (ESBLs).

Uses
- Surgical prophylaxis although 1st and 2nd generation cephalosporins are usually preferred
- Acute epiglottitis due to *Haemophilus influenzae*
- Empiric therapy of meningitis
- Intra-abdominal infections including peritonitis
- Community acquired and nosocomial pneumonia
- Urinary tract infections
- Sepsis of unknown origin

Contraindications
Hypersensitivity to cephalosporins
Serious penicillin hypersensitivity (10% cross-sensitivity)
Porphyria

Administration
- IV: 1 g 12 hourly, increased in life-threatening infections (e.g. meningitis) to 3 g 6 hourly

Reconstitute with 10 ml WFI, given over 3–5 min

Infection	Dose (g)	Interval (h)
Mild–moderate	1	12
Moderate–serious	2	8
Life–threatening	3	6

In severe renal impairment (<10 ml/min): halve dose

Adverse effects
Hypersensitivity
Transient ↑ LFTs
Clostridium difficile associated diarrhoea

Cautions
Concurrent use of nephrotoxic drugs (aminoglycosides, loop diuretics)
Severe renal impairment (halve dose)
False +ve urinary glucose (if tested for reducing substances)
False +ve Coombs' test

Organ failure
Renal: reduce dose

Renal replacement therapy
No further dose modification is required during renal replacement therapy

Used for treatment
of bacterial meningitis

CEFTAZIDIME

A third generation cephalosporin whose activity against Gram +ve organisms, most notably *S. aureus* is diminished in comparison with second generation cephalosporins, while action against Gram −ve organisms, including *Pseudomonas aeruginosa*, is enhanced. Ceftazidime is not active against enterococci, MRSA or *Bacteroides* spp.

Uses
Acute epiglottitis due to *Haemophilus influenzae*
Meningitis due to *Pseudomonas aeruginosa*
Intra-abdominal infections including peritonitis
Nosocomial pneumonia
Urinary tract infections
Severe sepsis of unknown origin
Febrile neutropenia

Contraindications
Hypersensitivity to cephalosporins
Serious penicillin hypersensitivity (10% cross-sensitivity)
Porphyria

Administration
• IV: 0.5–2 g 8–12 hourly depending on severity of infection

Reconstitute with 10 ml WFI, given over 3–5 min

Infection	Dose (g)	Interval (h)
Mild–moderate	0.5–1	12
Moderate–serious	1	8
Life-threatening	2	8

In renal impairment:

CC (ml/min)	Dose (g)	Interval (h)
20–50	1	8–12
10–20	1	12–24
<10	0.5	24–48

Adverse effects
Hypersensitivity
Transient ↑ LFTs
Clostridium difficile associated diarrhoea

Cautions

Renal impairment (reduce dose)

Concurrent use of nephrotoxic drugs (aminoglycosides, loop diuretics)

False +ve urinary glucose (if tested for reducing substances)

False +ve Coombs' test

Renal replacement therapy

Removed by HD/HF/PD, significant for high clearance techniques

For low clearance techniques dose as for CC <10 ml/min. If high clearance technique dose as for CC 10–20 ml/min

Levels can be monitored

CEFTRIAXONE

A third generation cephalosporin which is similar in many respects to cefotaxime, with enhanced activity against Gram −ve species in comparison to second generation cephalosporins. Ceftriaxone is not active against enterococci, MRSA, *Pseudomonas aeruginosa* or *Bacteroides* spp. Ceftriaxone has a prolonged serum half-life allowing for once daily dosing. However twice daily dosing is normally recommended for severe infections including meningitis.

Uses
- Surgical prophylaxis although 1st and 2nd generation cephalosporins are usually preferred
- Empiric therapy for meningitis
- Intra-abdominal infections including peritonitis
- Community acquired or nosocomial pneumonia
- Clearance of throat carriage in meningococcal disease

Contraindications
Hypersensitivity to cephalosporins
Serious penicillin hypersensitivity (10% cross-sensitivity)
Porphyria

Administration
- IV: 2 g once daily, increased to 2 g 12 hourly in severe infections

Reconstitute 2 g vial with 40 ml of 5% dextrose or 0.9% saline, given over at least 30 min

How not to use Ceftriaxone
Not to be dissolved in infusion fluids containing calcium (Hartmann's)

Adverse effects
Hypersensitivity
Transient ↑ liver enzymes
Clostridium difficile associated diarrhoea

CEFUROXIME

A second generation cephalosporin widely used in combination with metronidazole in the post-operative period following most abdominal procedures. Has greater activity against *Staphylococcus aureus* (including penicillinase-producing strains) compared with the third generation cephalosporins, but not active against MRSA, enterococcus, *Pseudomonas aeruginosa or Bacteroides* spp. It also has poor activity against penicillin resistant strains of *Streptococcus pneumoniae*.

Uses
- Surgical prophylaxis
- Acute epiglottitis due to *Haemophilus influenzae*
- Intra-abdominal infections including peritonitis
- Community acquired and nosocomial pneumonia
- Urinary tract infections
- Patients admitted from the community with sepsis of unknown origin
- Soft tissue infections

Contraindications
Hypersensitivity to cephalosporins
Serious penicillin hypersensitivity (10% cross-sensitivity)
Meningitis (high relapse rate)
Porphyria

Administration
- IV: 0.75–1.5 g 6–8 hourly

Reconstitute with 20 ml WFI, given over 3–5 min
In renal impairment:

CC (ml/min)	Dose (g)	Interval (h)
10–20	0.75	6–8
<10	0.75	8–12

Adverse effects
Hypersensitivity
Transient ↑ LFTs
Clostridium difficile associated diarrhoea

Cautions
Hypersensitivity to penicillins
Renal impairment

Renal replacement therapy
Removed by HD/HF/PD but significant only for high clearance techniques. Dose for high clearance renal replacement 750 mg 12 hourly. For low clearance techniques dose as for CC <10 ml/min

CIPROFLOXACIN

Ciprofloxacin is a fluoroquinolone with bactericidal activity against *E.coli,* *Klebsiella* spp., *Proteus* spp., *Serratia* spp., *Salmonella* spp., *Campylobacter* spp., *Pseudomonas aeruginosa, Haemophilus influenzae, Neisseria* spp. *and* *Staphylococcus* spp. Many strains of MRSA in the UK are resistant and the use of ciprofloxacin may be associated with increased rates of MRSA colonisation. Activity against many other Gram +ve organisms is poor.

Uses
Respiratory tract infection – avoid if possibility of pneumococcal infection
Severe urinary tract infection
Intra-abdominal infections
Meningitis prophylaxis (unlicensed)
Severely ill patients with gastroenteritis
Suspected enteric fever
Sepsis of unknown origin

Administration
• For infection

IV infusion: 200–400 mg 12 hourly, given over 30–60 min

8 hourly dosing may be required for *P. aeruginosa* and other less susceptible Gram −ve organisms

Available in 100 ml bottle containing 200 mg ciprofloxacin in 0.9% saline and 200 ml bottle containing 400 mg ciprofloxacin in 0.9% saline. Contains Na$^+$ 15.4 mmol/100 ml bottle.

Also available in 100 ml bag containing 200 mg ciprofloxacin in 5% dextrose and 200 ml bottle containing 400 mg ciprofloxacin in 5% dextrose.

Oral: 500–750 mg 12 hourly

In severe renal impairment (serum creatinine >265 μmol/L or creatinine clearance <20 ml/min, the total daily dose may be reduced by half.

• Meningitis prophylaxis

Oral: 500 mg as a single dose or 12 hourly for two days
Child 5–12 years: 250 mg orally, as a single dose

How not to use ciprofloxacin
Do not put in fridge (crystal formation)
Do not use as sole agent where pneumococcal infection likely

Adverse effects
Transient increases in bilirubin, liver enzymes and creatinine
Tendon damage and rupture, especially in the elderly and those taking corticosteroids (may occur within 48 hours)

C

Cautions
Concurrent administration with theophylline (increased plasma level of theophylline)
Concurrent administration with cyclosporin (transient increase in serum creatinine)
Epilepsy (increased risk of fits)
Concurrent administration of corticosteroids (risk of tendon damage and rupture)

Organ failure
Renal: reduce dose

Renal replacement therapy
No further dose modification is required during renal replacement therapy

CIPROFLOXACIN

CLARITHROMYCIN

Clarithromycin is an erythromycin derivative with slightly greater activity, a longer half-life and higher tissue penetration than erythromycin. Adverse effects are thought to be less common than with erythromycin. Resistance rates in Gram +ve organisms limit its use for severe soft tissue infections.

Uses
Community acquired pneumonia
Infective exacerbations of COPD
Pharyngeal and sinus infections
Soft tissue infections

Administration
- Orally: 250–500 mg 12 hourly
- IV: 500 mg 12 hourly

Reconstitute in 10 ml WFI. Then make up to 250 ml with 5% dextrose or 0.9% saline and give over 60 min
If creatinine clearance <30 ml/min, give half the dose (250 mg 12 hourly)

How not to use clarithromycin
Should not be given as IV bolus or IM injection

Adverse effects
Gastrointestinal intolerance
↑ LFTs (usually reversible)

Organ failure
Renal: reduce dose

250mls Normal Saline

espiratory-tract infections, mild to moderate
in & soft tissue
fections, otitis media, Helicobacter pylori
eradication

HANDBOOK OF DRUGS IN INTENSIVE CARE

CLOMETHIAZOLE C

Clomethiazole is available as capsules (192 mg) and syrup (250 mg/5 ml), but no longer available as a 0.8% solution for IV use. One capsule is equivalent to 5 ml syrup. The capsule contains 192 mg clomethiazole (base) while the syrup contains 250 mg clomethiazole edisilate per 5 ml. The difference in weight is due to the inactive edisilate group.

Uses
Alcohol withdrawal
Restlessness and agitation

Contraindications
Alcohol-dependent patients who continue to drink

Administration
1 capsule ≡ 5 ml syrup

- Alcohol withdrawal

Oral: Day 1 9–12 capsules in 3–4 divided doses

Day 2 6–8 capsules in 3–4 divided doses

Day 3 4–6 capsules in 3–4 divided doses

Then gradually reduce over days 4–6

Do not treat for >9 days

- Restlessness and agitation

Oral: 1 capsule 3 times daily

How not to use clomethiazole
Prolonged use (risk of dependence)
Abrupt withdrawal

Adverse effects
Increased nasopharyngeal and bronchial secretions
Conjunctival irritation
Headache

Cautions
Concurrent use of other CNS depressants will produce excessive sedation
Cardiac and respiratory disease – confusion may indicate hypoxia
Hepatic impairment – sedation can mask hepatic coma
Renal impairment

Organ failure
Hepatic: Reduced clearance with accumulation. Can precipitate coma
Renal: Increase cerebral sensitivity

CLONIDINE

Clonidine is an α_2 adrenoceptor agonist which may have a protective effect on cardiovascular morbidity and mortality in the critically ill patient. The mechanism of the protective effect is likely to be manifold. α_2 adrenoceptor agonists attenuate haemodynamic instability, inhibit central sympathetic discharge, reduce peripheral norepinephrine release, and dilate post-stenotic coronary vessels. Its use as an antihypertensive agent has since been superseded by other drugs. It has a useful sedative property, which is synergistic with opioids and other sedative agents. It is a useful short-term adjuvant to sedation especially following extubation where there is a high sympathetic drive and in the agitated patient. Its usage should not exceed 3 days, as withdrawal can lead to rebound hypertension and agitation.

Uses
Short-term adjunct to sedation

Contraindications
Hypotension
Porphyria

Administration
- IV bolus: 50 microgram 8 hourly, given slowly over 10–15 min, may be increased gradually to 250 microgram 8 hourly
- IV infusion: 30–50 microgram/h

Oral: 50 microgram 8 hourly, may be increased gradually to 400 microgram 8 hourly

Compatible with 5% dextrose and 0.9% saline

How not to use clonidine
Sudden withdrawal if used for longer than 3 days

Adverse effects
Bradycardia
Hypotension
Fluid retention
Dry mouth
Sedation
Depression
Constipation

Cautions

Avoid prolong use and sudden withdrawal (rebound hypertension)

Peripheral vascular disease (concomitant use with beta blockers may worsen condition)

2nd degree heart block (may progress to complete heart block)

Avoid concomitant use with:

Beta blockers (bradycardia)

Tricyclics (counteract effect)

NSAIDs (sodium and water retention)

Digoxin (bradycardia)

Haloperidol (prolongation of QT interval)

Organ failure

Renal: reduce dose

CLONIDINE

CLOPIDOGREL

In addition to standard therapy (aspirin, LMWH, β-blocker and nitrate), clopidogrel reduces the risk of MI, stroke and cardiovascular death in patients with unstable angina and non–ST-elevation MI (The CURE investigators. *N Eng J Med* 2001; **345:** 494–502). NICE and the European Society of Cardiology both endorse the use of clopidogrel in combination with aspirin in non–ST-elevation acute coronary syndrome patients.

Uses
Acute coronary syndrome

Contraindications
Warfarin
Severe liver impairment
Active bleeding
Breast feeding

Administration
Unstable angina and non–ST-elevation MI: single 300 mg loading dose, followed by 75 mg daily (with aspirin 75 mg/day) for up to 12 months

Monitor: FBC
Clotting screen

Discontinue 7 days prior to surgery

How not to use clopidogrel
Omit clopidogrel if patient likely to go for CABG within 5 days
Not recommended under 18 years of age
Pregnancy

Adverse effects
Bleeding
Abnormal LFTs and raised serum creatinine
Haematological disorders including pancytopenia

Cautions
Avoid for first few days after MI and for 7 days after ischaemic stroke
Increase risk of bleeding with the concurrent use of:
Aspirin (although recommended for up to 12 months in CURE study)
NSAIDs
Heparin
Thrombolytics
Glycoprotein IIb/IIIa inhibitors

Organ failure
Hepatic: avoid in severe liver impairment

CO-AMOXICLAV

Amoxycillin + clavulanic acid (β–lactamase inhibitor). The β–lactamase inhibitory action of clavulinic acid extends the spectrum of antibacterial activity of amoxycillin.

Uses
Respiratory tract infections
Genito-urinary tract infections
Intra-abdominal sepsis
Surgical prophylaxis

Contraindications
Penicillin hypersensitivity

Administration
• IV: 1.2 g 8 hourly (6 hourly in severe infections)

Reconstitute with 20 ml WFI, given IV over 3–5 min
In renal impairment:
Initial dose of 1.2 g, then:

CC (ml/min)	Dose (g)	Interval (h)
10–20	0.6	12
<10	0.6	24

How not to use co-amoxiclav
Do not mix with aminoglycoside in same syringe (will inactivate aminoglycoside)

Adverse effects
Hypersensitivity
Cholestatic jaundice (usually self-limiting)
Bleeding and prothrombin time may be prolonged

Organ failure
Renal: reduce dose

Renal replacement therapy
Removed by HD/HF/PD but significant only for high clearance techniques. Dose as for CC 10–20 ml/min. Pharmacokinetics of the amoxycillin and clauvulanic acid are closely matched, probably cleared at similar rates.

Kept in CD cupboard

HDU Key

CODEINE PHOSPHATE

Codeine has a low affinity for the μ and k opioid receptors. It is relatively more effective when given orally than parenterally. It is useful as an antitussive and for the treatment of diarrhoea. Side-effects are uncommon and respiratory depression is seldom a problem. This explains its traditional use to provide analgesia for head-injured and neurosurgical patients. Doses >60 mg do not improve analgesic activity but may increase side-effects. Of it, 10% undergoes demethylation to morphine – this possibly contributing to the analgesic effect.

Uses
Mild to moderate pain
Diarrhoea and excessive ileostomy output
Antitussive

Contraindications
Airway obstruction

Administration
- Orally: 30–60 mg 4–6 hourly
- IM: 30–60 mg 4–6 hourly

How not to use codeine phosphate
Not for IV use

Adverse effects
Drowsiness
Constipation
Nausea and vomiting
Respiratory depression

Cautions
Enhanced sedative and respiratory depression from interaction with:

- benzodiazepines
- antidepressants
- anti-psychotics

MAOI (hypertension, hyperpyrexia, convulsions and coma)
Head injury and neurosurgical patients (may exacerbate ↑ ICP as a result of ↑ $PaCO_2$)
May cause renal failure

Organ failure
CNS: sedative effects increased
Hepatic: can precipitate coma
Renal: increase cerebral sensitivity

Renal replacement therapy
No further dose modification is required during renal replacement therapy

CO-TRIMOXAZOLE

Sulphamethoxazole and trimethoprim are used in combination because of their synergistic activity. Increasing resistance to sulphonamides and the high incidence of sulphonamide-related side-effects have diminished the value of co-trimoxazole. Trimethoprim alone is now preferred for urinary tract infections and exacerbations of chronic bronchitis. However, high-dose co-trimoxazole is the preferred treatment for *Pneumocystis carinii* pneumonia (PCP). It has certain theoretical advantages over pentamidine: pentamidine accumulates slowly in the lung parenchyma and improvement may occur more slowly, co-trimoxazole has a broad-spectrum of activity and may treat any bacterial co-pathogens. Pneumonia caused by *Pneumocystis carinii* (now renamed *Pneumocystis jirovecii*) occurs in immunosuppressed patients; it is a common cause of pneumonia in AIDS. High dose co-trimoxazole with corticosteroid therapy is the treatment of choice for moderate to severe infections. Co-trimoxazole prophylaxis should be considered for severely immunocompromised patients.

Uses
Pneumocystis carinii pneumonia

Contraindications
Pregnancy
Severe renal/hepatic failure
Blood disorders
Porphyria

Administration
* *Pneumocystis carinii* pneumonia

60 mg/kg 12 hourly IV for 14 days followed orally for a further 7 days
IV infusion: dilute every 1 ml (96 mg) in 25 ml 5% dextrose or 0.9% saline, given over 1.5–2 h. If fluid restriction necessary, dilute in half the amount of 5% dextrose
Adjuvant corticosteroid has been shown to improve survival. The steroid should be started at the same time as the co-trimoxazole and should be withdrawn before the antibiotic treatment is complete. Oral prednisolone 50–80 mg daily or IV hydrocortisone 100 mg 6 hourly or IV dexamethasone 8 mg 6 hourly or IV methylprednisolone 1 g for 5 days, then dose reduced to complete 21 days of treatment.

* PCP prophylaxis

Oral: 960 mg daily or 960 mg on alternate days (3 times a week) or 480 mg daily to improve tolerance
In renal impairment (CC <20 ml/min): reduce dose to 75%
Note: treatment should be stopped if rashes or serious blood disorders develop. A fall in white cell count should be treated with folic/folinic acid and a dose reduction to 75%.

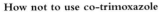

C

How not to use co-trimoxazole

Concurrent use of co-trimoxazole and pentamidine is not of benefit and may increase the incidence of serious side-effects.

Adverse effects

Nausea, vomiting and diarrhoea (including pseudomembranous colitis)
Rashes (including Stevens–Johnson syndrome)
Blood disorders (includes leucopenia, thrombocytopenia, anaemia)
Fluid overload (due to large volumes required)

Cautions

Elderly
Renal impairment (rashes and blood disorders increase, may cause further deterioration in renal function)

Renal replacement therapy

Removed by HD/HF but significant only with high clearance techniques. Give 30 mg twice a day (or 60 mg once a day) if low clearance technique or 60 mg twice a day for 3 days followed by 30 mg twice a day (or 60 mg once a day) if high clearance technique. Plasma levels of sulphamethoxazole and trimethoprim can be measured and are useful in renal failure and support. Not significantly removed by PD

CYCLIZINE

Anti-histamine with antimuscarinic effects.

Uses
Nausea and vomiting

Administration
• IM/IV: 50 mg 8 hourly

Adverse effects
Anticholinergic: drowsiness, dryness of mouth, blurred vision, tachycardia

Cautions
Sedative effect enhanced by concurrent use of other CNS depressants

Organ failure
CNS: sedative effects enhanced

Give slowly.

Pt can become tachycardiac
if given too quickly

CICLOSPORIN

Ciclosporin is a cyclic peptide molecule derived from a soil fungus. It is a potent nephrotoxin, producing interstitial renal fibrosis with tubular atrophy. Monitoring of cyclosporin blood level is essential.
Normal range: 100–300 microgram/l
For renal transplants: lower end of range
For heart/lung/liver: upper end of range

Uses
Prevention of organ rejection after transplantation

Administration
• IV dose: 1–5 mg/kg/day

To be diluted 1 in 20 to 1 in 100 with 0.9% saline or 5% dextrose
To be given over 2–6 h
Infusion should be completed within 12 h if using PVC lines
Switch to oral for long-term therapy

• Oral: 1.5 times IV dose given 12 hourly
Monitor:
Hepatic function
Renal function
Cyclosporin blood level (pre-dose sample)

How not to use ciclosporin
Must not be given as IV bolus
Do not infuse at >12 h if using PVC lines – leaching of phthalates from the PVC

Adverse effects
Enhanced renal sensitivity to insults
↑ Plasma urea and serum creatinine secondary to glomerulosclerosis
Hypertension – responds to conventional antihypertensives
Hepatocellular damage (↑ transaminases)
Hyperuricaemia
Gingival hypertrophy
Hirsuitism
Tremors or seizures at high serum levels

Cautions
↑ susceptibility to infections and lymphoma
↑ nephrotoxic effects with concurrent use of other nephrotoxic drugs

DALTEPARIN (Fragmin)

A low molecular weight heparin (LMWH) with greater anti-Factor Xa activity than anti-IIa (antithrombin) activity, which theoretically makes it more effective at preventing thrombin formation than standard (unfractionated) heparin with an equal anti-Factor Xa and anti-IIa ratio.

After SC injection, LMWHs are better absorbed than unfractionated heparin, and bind less to proteins in plasma and in the endothelial wall. As a result they have around 90% bioavailability compared to 10–30% with unfractionated heparin. After SC injection, the plasma half-life of LMWHs is around 4 hours, enabling a single dose to provide effective anti-coagulant activity for up to 24 hours the treatment of venous thromboembolism peri- and post-operative surgical thomboprophy-laxis, and the prevention of clotting in the extra corporeal circulation during haemodialysis or haemofiltration.

The incidence of bleeding is similar between LMWHs and unfractionated heparin. Both can cause thrombocytopenia – the incidence of immune-mediated thrombocytopenia is about 2–3% of patients treated with unfrac-tionated heparin, typically developing after 5–10 days' treatment. In clinical trials with dalteparin, thrombocytopenia occurred in up to 1% of patients receiving treatment for unstable angina, undergoing abdominal surgery or hip replacement surgery. LMWHs are at least as well tolerated and effective as unfractionated heparin in the treatment of venous thromboembolism. They simplify treatment (once daily dosing, no IV cannulation) and require less monitoring by blood tests than unfractionated heparin.

Uses
Peri- and post-operative surgical thomboprophylaxis
Treatment of DVT and pulmonary embolism or both
Unstable angina
Prevention of clotting in extracorporeal circuits

Contraindications
Generalised bleeding tendencies
Acute GI ulcer
Cerebral haemorrhage
Sub-acute endocarditis
Heparin induced immune thrombocytopenia
Injuries to and operations on the CNS, eyes and ears
Known haemorrhagic diathesis
Hypersensitivity to Fragmin or other LMWHs and/or heparins

Administration

- Peri- and post-operative surgical prophylaxis – moderate risk
  2,500 units only daily SC
- Peri- and post-operative surgical prophylaxis – high risk
  5,000 units only daily SC
- Treatment of DVT and pulmonary embolus or both
  - Start dalteparin with oral warfarin (as soon as possible) until pro-thrombin time in therapeutic range.
  - 200 units/kg once daily SC up to maximum daily dose of 18,000 units or 100 units/kg twice daily if increased risk of haemorrhage.

Body weight (kg)	Dose (200 units/kg)
<46	7,500 once daily SC
46–56	10,000 once daily SC
57–68	12,500 once daily SC
69–82	15,000 once daily SC
≥83	18,000 once daily SC

- Unstable angina
  Acute phase: 120 units/kg 12 hourly SC
  Maximum dose: 10,000 units twice daily
  Concomitant treatment with low dose aspirin
  Recommended treatment period up to 8 days
  - Extended phase: Men <70 kg, 5,000 units once daily SC, >70 kg 7,500 units once daily SC
  - Women <80 kg 5,000 units once daily SC, >80 kg 7,500 units once daily SC

  Treatment should not be given for more than 45 days.

Monitor: platelets
APTT monitoring is not usually required

In overdose, 100 units dalteparin is inhibited by 1 mg protamine

Adverse effects

Subcutaneous haematoma at injection site
Bleeding at high doses, e.g., anti-Factor Xa levels greater than 1.5 iu/ml, however at recommended doses bleeding rarely occurs
Transient increase in liver enzymes (ALT) but no clinical significance has been demonstrated
Rarely thrombocytopenia

DANTROLENE

D

Dantrolene is thought to work in MH by interfering with the release of calcium from sarcoplasmic reticulum to the myoplasm. The average dose required to reverse the manifestations of MH is 2.5 mg/kg. If a relapse or recurrence occurs, dantrolene should be re-administered at the last effective dose. When used for the short-term treatment of MH there are usually no side-effects. Dantrolene has been used in the treatment of hyperthermia and rhabdomyolysis caused by theophylline overdose, consumption of 'Ecstasy' and 'Eve', and in the neuroleptic malignant syndrome and thyrotoxic storm. Neuroleptic malignant syndrome is characterized by hyperthermia, muscle rigidity, tachycardia, labile BP, sweating, autonomic dysfunction, urinary incontinence and fluctuating level of consciousness. It has been reported with haloperidol, fluphenazine, chlorpromazine, droperidol, thioridazine, metoclopramide, flupenthixol decanoate and tricyclic antidepressants.

Uses
MH (p. 202)
Neuroleptic malignant syndrome (unlicensed)
Thyrotoxic storm (unlicensed)
Hyperthermia and rhabdomyolysis associated with theophylline overdose, consumption of 'Ecstasy' and 'Eve' (unlicensed)

Contraindications
Hepatic impairment (worsens)

Administration
• IV: 1 mg/kg, repeated PRN up to 10 mg/kg

Reconstitute each 20 mg vial with 60 ml WFI and shaken well
Each vial contains a mixture of 20 mg dantrolene sodium, 3 g mannitol and sodium hydroxide to yield a pH 9.5 when reconstituted with 60 ml WFI

Adverse effects
Rash
Diarrhoea
Muscle weakness
Hepatotoxicity

Cautions
Concurrent use of diltiazem (arrhythmias)
Concurrent use of calcium channel blockers (hypotension, myocardial depression and hyperkalaemia reported with verapamil)

DESMOPRESSIN (DDAVP)

Pituitary diabetes insipidus (DI) results from a deficiency of antidiuretic hormone (ADH) secretion. Desmopressin is an analogue of ADH. Treatment may be required for a limited period only in DI following head trauma or pituitary surgery. It is also used in the differential diagnosis of DI. Restoration of the ability to concentrate urine after water deprivation confirms a diagnosis of pituitary DI. Failure to respond occurs in nephrogenic DI.

Uses
Pituitary DI – diagnosis and treatment

Administration
• Diagnosis

Intranasally: 20 microgram
SC/IM: 2 microgram

• Treatment

Intranasally: 5–20 microgram once or twice daily
SC/IM/IV: 1–4 microgram daily
Monitor fluid intake
Patient should be weighed daily

Adverse effects
Fluid retention
Hyponatraemia
Headache
Nausea and vomiting

Cautions
Renal impairment
Cardiac disease
Hypertension
Cystic fibrosis

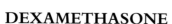

DEXAMETHASONE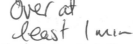

Dexamethasone has very high glucocorticoid activity and insignificant mineralocorticoid activity, making it particularly suitable for conditions where water retention would be a disadvantage. Adjuvant corticosteroid has been shown to improve survival in *Pneumocystis carinii* pneumonia.

Uses
Cerebral oedema
Laryngeal oedema
Adjunct in *Pneumocystis carinii* pneumonia (see co-trimoxazole and pentamidine)
Bacterial meningitis, particularly where pneumococcal suspected

Contraindications
Systemic infection (unless specific anti-microbial therapy given)

Administration
- Cerebral oedema

IV bolus: 8 mg initially, then 4 mg 6 hourly as required for 2–10 days

- *Pneumocystis carinii* pneumonia

IV bolus: 8 mg 6 hourly 5 days, then dose reduced to complete 21 days of treatment
The steroid should be started at the same time as the co-trimoxazole or pentamidine and should be withdrawn before the antibiotic treatment is complete.

How not to use dexamethasone
Do not stop abruptly after prolonged use (adrenocortical insufficiency)

Adverse effects
Perineal irritation may follow IV administration of the phosphate ester
Prolonged use may also lead to the following problems:

- Increased susceptibility to infections
- Impaired wound healing
- Peptic ulceration
- Muscle weakness (proximal myopathy)
- Osteoporosis
- Hyperglycaemia

Cautions
Diabetes mellitus
Concurrent use of NSAID (increased risk of GI bleeding)

DIAZEPAM

Available formulated in either propylene glycol or a lipid emulsion (diazemul) which causes minimal thrombophlebitis. Also available in a rectal solution (stesolid) which takes up to 10 min to work.

Uses
Termination of epileptic fit

Contraindications
Airway obstruction

Administration
- IV: diazemuls 5–10 mg over 2 min, repeated if necessary after 15 min, up to total 30 mg
- PR: stesolid up to 20 mg

How not to use diazepam
IM injection – painful and unpredictable absorption

Adverse effects
Respiratory depression and apnoea
Drowsiness
Hypotension and bradycardia

Cautions
Airway obstruction with further neurological damage
Enhanced and prolonged sedative effect in the elderly
Additive effects with other CNS depressants

Organ failure
CNS: enhanced and prolonged sedative effect
Respiratory: ↑ respiratory depression
Hepatic: enhanced and prolonged sedative effect. Can precipitate coma
Renal: enhanced and prolonged sedative effect

Renal replacement therapy
No further dose modification is required during renal replacement therapy

DICLOFENAC

NSAID with analgesic, anti-inflammatory and antipyretic properties. It has an opioid-sparing effect. In the critically ill, the side-effects of NSAID are such that they have to be used with extreme caution – especially where there is a risk of stress ulceration, and renal impairment and bleeding diatheses are common. Ensure patient is adequately hydrated.

Uses
Pain, especially musculoskeletal
Antipyretic (unlicensed)

Contraindications
Uncontrolled asthma
Hypersensitivity to aspirin and other NSAID (cross sensitivity)
Active peptic ulceration (bleeding)
Haemophilia and other clotting disorders (bleeding)
Renal and hepatic impairment (worsens)
Hypovolaemia

Administration
• Pain

PO/NG: 50 mg 8 hourly
PR: 100 mg suppository 18 hourly
IV infusion: 75 mg diluted with 100–500 ml 0.9% saline or 5% dextrose. Buffer the solution with sodium bicarbonate (0.5 ml 8.4% or 1 ml 4.2%)
Give over 30–120 min
Once prepared use immediately
Maximum daily dose: 150 mg

• Antipyretic

IV bolus: 10 mg diluted with 20 ml 0.9% saline, given over 3 min

How not to use diclofenac
Do not give suppository in inflammatory bowel disease affecting anus, rectum and sigmoid colon (worsening of disease)

Adverse effects
Epigastric pain
Peptic ulcer
Rashes
Worsening of liver function tests
Prolonged bleeding time (platelet dysfunction)
Acute renal failure – in patients with:

• pre-existing renal and hepatic impairment

• hypovolaemia

• renal hypoperfusion

• sepsis

D

Cautions
Elderly
Hypovolaemia
Renal and hepatic impairment
Previous peptic ulceration

Organ failure
Hepatic: worsens
Renal: worsens

DICLOFENAC

DIGOXIN

D

A cardiac glycoside with both anti-arrhythmic and inotropic properties. Digoxin is useful for controlling the ventricular response in AF and atrial flutter.

Heart failure may also be improved. It is principally excreted unchanged by the kidney and will therefore accumulate in renal impairment.

Uses
SVT

Contraindications
Intermittent complete heart block
Second-degree AV block
WPW syndrome
Hypertrophic obstructive cardiomyopathy
Constrictive pericarditis

Administration
- IV loading dose: 0.5–1.0 mg in 50 ml 5% dextrose or 0.9% saline, given over 2 h
- Maintenance dose: 62.5–500 microgram daily (renal function is the most important determinant of maintenance dosage)

Monitor:
- ECG
- Serum digoxin level (p. 193)

How not to use digoxin
IM injections not recommended

Adverse effects
Anorexia, nausea, vomiting
Diarrhoea, abdominal pain
Visual disturbances, headache
Fatigue, drowsiness, confusion, delirium, hallucinations
Arrhythmias – all forms
Heart block

DIGOXIN

D

DIGOXIN

Cautions

Absorption from oral administration reduced by sucralfate and ion-exchange resins, cholestyramine and colestipol

Hypokalaemia and hypomagnesaemia increases the sensitivity to digoxin, and the following drugs may predispose to toxicity:

- Amphotericin
- β_2 sympathomimetics
- Corticosteroids
- Loop diuretics
- Thiazides

Hypercalcaemia is inhibitory to the positive inotropic action of digoxin and potentiates the toxic effects:

Plasma concentration of digoxin increased by:

- Amiodarone
- Diltiazem
- Nicardipine
- Propafenone
- Quinidine
- Verapamil

Digoxin toxicity (DC shock may cause fatal ventricular arrhythmia) – stop digoxin at least 24 h before cardioversion

β-Blockers and verapamil increase AV block and bradycardia

Suxamethonium predisposes to arrhythmias

Organ failure

Renal: toxicity – reduce dose

Renal replacement therapy

Removed by HD/HF but significant only with high clearance techniques. Dose according to measured plasma levels. With high clearance levels likely dose needed 125–250 microgram per day, 62.5 microgram per day or less with low clearance technique. Not significantly removed by PD

DOBUTAMINE

D

Dobutamine has predominant β_1 effects that increases heart rate and force of contraction. It also has mild β_2 and α_1 effects and decreases peripheral and pulmonary vascular resistance. Systolic BP may be increased because of the augmented cardiac output. Dobutamine has no specific effects on renal or splanchnic blood flow, but may increase renal blood flow due to an increase in cardiac output.

Uses
Low cardiac output states

Contraindications
Before adequate intravascular volume replacement
Idiopathic hypertrophic subaortic stenosis

Administration
• IV infusion: 1–25 microgram/kg/min via a central vein

Titrate dose according to HR, BP, cardiac output, presence of ectopic beats and urine output
250 mg made up to 50 ml 5% dextrose or 0.9% saline (5000 microgram/ml)

Dosage chart (ml/h)

Weight (kg)	Dose (microgram/kg/min)					
	2.5	5.0	7.5	10	15	20
50	1.5	3.0	4.5	6.0	9.0	12.0
60	1.8	3.6	5.4	7.2	10.8	14.5
70	2.1	4.2	6.3	8.4	12.75	16.8
80	2.4	4.8	7.2	9.6	14.4	19.2
90	2.7	5.4	8.1	10.8	16.2	21.6
100	3.0	6.0	9.0	12.0	18.0	24.0
110	3.3	6.6	9.9	13.2	19.8	26.4
120	3.6	7.2	10.8	14.4	21.6	28.8

DOBUTAMINE

D

How not to use dobutamine
In the absence of invasive cardiac monitoring
Inadequate correction of hypovolaemia before starting dobutamine
Do not connect to CVP lumen used for monitoring pressure (surge of drug during flushing of line)
Incompatible with alkaline solutions, e.g. sodium bicarbonate, frusemide, phenytoin and enoximone

Adverse effects
Tachycardia
Ectopic beats

Cautions
Acute myocardial ischaemia or MI
β-Blockers (may cause dobutamine to be less effective)

DOPAMINE

D

A naturally occurring catecholamine that acts directly on α, β_1 and dopaminergic receptors and indirectly by releasing noradrenaline.

- At low doses (0.5–2.5 microgram/kg/min) it increases renal and mesenteric blood flow by stimulating dopamine receptors. The ↑ renal blood flow results in ↑ GFR and ↑ renal sodium excretion
- Doses between 2.5 and 10 microgram/kg/min stimulates β_1 receptors causing ↑ myocardial contractility, stroke volume and cardiac output
- Doses >10 microgram/kg/min stimulate a receptors causing ↑ SVR, ↓ renal blood flow and ↑ potential for arrhythmias

The distinction between dopamine's predominant dopaminergic and β effects at low doses and α effects at higher doses is not helpful in clinical practice due to marked interindividual variation.

Uses
Low dose to maintain urine output
Septic shock
Low cardiac output

Contraindications
Attempt to increase urine output in patients inadequately fluid resuscitated
Phaeochromocytoma
Tachyarrhythmias or VF

Administration
- Low dose: 0.5–2.5 microgram/kg/min to produce renal vasodilatation
- Larger doses: 2.5–10 microgram/kg/min to increase cardiac contractility
- Doses >10 microgram/kg/min stimulates α-receptors and may cause renal vasoconstriction

200 mg made up to 50 ml 5% dextrose or 0.9% saline (4000 microgram/ml)
Dosage chart (ml/h)

DOPAMINE

Weight (kg)	Dose (microgram/kg/min)				
	2.5	5.0	7.5	10	15
50	1.9	3.8	5.6	7.5	11.3
60	2.3	4.5	6.8	9.0	13.5
70	2.6	5.3	7.9	10.5	15.8
80	3.0	6.0	9.0	12.0	18.0
90	3.4	6.8	10.1	13.5	20.3
100	3.8	7.5	11.3	15	22.5
110	4.1	8.3	12.4	16.5	24.8
120	4.5	9.0	13.5	18.0	27.0

D

Give via a central vein via accurate infusion pump
Reduce dosage if urine output decreases or there is increasing tachy-cardia or development of new arrhythmias

How not to use dopamine
Do not use a peripheral vein (risk of extravasation)
Do not connect to CVP lumen used for monitoring pressure (surge of drug during flushing of line)
Incompatible with alkaline solutions, e.g. sodium bicarbonate, frusemide, phenytoin and enoximone
Discard solution if cloudy, discoloured, or >24 h old

Adverse effects
Ectopic beats
Tachycardia
Angina
Gut ischaemia
Vasoconstriction

Cautions
MAOI (reduce dose by one-tenth of usual dose)
Peripheral vascular disease (monitor any changes in colour or tempera-ture of the skin of the extremities)
If extravasation of dopamine occurs – phentolamine 10 mg in 15 ml 0.9% saline should be infiltrated into the ischaemic area with a 23-G needle

Organ failure
May accumulate in septic shock because of ↓ hepatic function

DOPEXAMINE

D

Dopexamine is the synthetic analogue of dopamine. It has potent β_2 activity with one-third the potency of dopamine on dopamine 1 receptor. There is no a activity. Dopexamine increases HR and CO, causes peripheral vasodilatation, ↑ renal and splanchnic blood flow, and ↓ PCWP. Current interest in dopexamine is centred on its dopaminergic and anti-inflammatory activity. The anti-inflammatory activity and improved splanchnic blood flow may be due to dopexamine's β_2 rather than DA 1 effect. The usual dose for its anti-inflammatory activity and to improve renal, mesenteric, splanchnic and hepatic blood flow is between 0.25 and 0.5 microgram/kg/min. In comparison with other inotropes, dopexamine causes less increase in myocardial oxygen consumption.

Uses
To improve renal, mesenteric, splanchnic and hepatic blood flow
Short-term treatment of acute heart failure

Contraindications
Concurrent MAOI administration
Left ventricular outlet obstruction (HOCM, aortic stenosis)
Phaeochromocytoma

Administration
Correction of hypovolaemia before starting dopexamine

- Dose: start at 0.25 microgram/kg/min, increasing up to 6 microgram/kg/min

Titrate according to patient's response: HR, rhythm, BP, urine output and, whenever possible, cardiac output
50 mg made up to 50 ml 5% dextrose or 0.9% saline (1000 microgram/ml)
Dosage chart (ml/h)

Weight (kg)	Dose (microgram/kg/min)				
	0.25	0.5	1	2	3
50	0.8	1.5	3.0	6.0	9.0
60	0.9	1.8	3.6	7.2	10.8
70	1.1	2.1	4.2	8.4	12.6
80	1.2	2.4	4.8	9.6	14.4
90	1.4	2.7	5.4	10.8	16.2
100	1.5	3.0	6.0	12.0	18.0
110	1.7	3.3	6.6	13.2	19.8
120	1.8	3.6	7.2	14.4	21.6

D

How not to use dopexamine
Do not connect to CVP lumen used for monitoring pressure (surge of drug during flushing of line)
Incompatible with alkaline solutions, e.g. sodium bicarbonate, frusemide, phenytoin and enoximone

Adverse effects
Dose-related increases in HR
Hypotension
Angina
Hypokalaemia
Hyperglycaemia

Cautions
Thrombocytopenia (a further decrease may occur)
IHD (especially following acute MI)

DROPERIDOL

A butyrophenone with useful anti-emetic properties even at a fraction of the usual neuroleptic dose.

Uses
Nausea and vomiting

Contraindications
Parkinson's disease

Administration
- IV bolus: 0.625–1.25 mg
- Added to PCAS pumps: 5 mg in 60 mg morphine

Adverse effects
Drowsiness, apathy, nightmares
Extra-pyramidal movements

Cautions
Concurrent use of other CNS depressants (enhanced sedation)

Organ failure
CNS: sedative effects increased
Hepatic: can precipitate coma
Renal: increased cerebral sensitivity

Renal replacement therapy
No further dose modification is required during renal replacement therapy

DROTRECOGIN ALFA (Activated)

Drotrecogin alfa (*Xigris*) is indicated for the treatment of adult patients with severe sepsis with multiple organ failure when added to best standard care. Treatment should be started within 48 hours, and preferably within 24 hours, of onset of the first documented sepsis-induced organ dysfunction. The recommended dose of *Xigris* is 24 microgram/kg/hr given as a continuous intravenous infusion for a total duration of 96 hours. No dose adjustment is required in adult patients with severe sepsis with regard to age, gender, hepatic or renal function.

Uses
Severe sepsis with multiple organ failure

Contraindications
- Active internal bleeding; patients at increased risk for bleeding; platelet count <30,000 × 10^6/l, even if the platelet count is increased after transfusions; known bleeding diathesis except for acute coagulopathy related to sepsis; any major surgery; patients with epidural catheter; history of severe head trauma; gastro-intestinal bleeding within 6 weeks; trauma patients at increased risk of bleeding

- Patients with intracranial pathology; neoplasm or evidence of cerebral herniation; haemorrhagic stroke within 3 months; A-V malformations

- Concurrent heparin therapy ≥15 International Units/kg/hour

- Chronic severe hepatic disease

See appendix H

Administration
See appendixes I and J

How not to use drotrecogin alfa
Xigris should not be used in patients with single organ dysfunction or a low risk of death (APACHE II score <25)

Adverse effects
Bleeding

- *Serious Bleeding Events During the Infusion Period*

Incidence of serious bleeding events 2.4%
Incidence of CNS bleeds 0.3%
Recent surgery was associated with a higher risk of serious bleeding

- *Serious Bleeding Events During the 28-Day Study Period*

Incidence serious bleeding events 3.5%
Incidence of CNS bleeds 0.2%

D

Cautions

- Recent administration of thrombolytic therapy, oral anticoagulants, aspirin or other platelet inhibitors, or recent ischaemic stroke, the risks of the administration of *Xigris* should be weighed against the anticipated benefits. No observed increase in the risk of bleeding events was reported as serious adverse events in drotrecogin alfa (activated) patients receiving prophylactic doses of unfractionated or low molecular weight heparin

- For procedures with an inherent bleeding risk, discontinue *Xigris* for 2 hours prior to the start of the procedure. *Xigris* may be restarted 12 hours after major invasive procedures

- If sequential tests of haemostasis (including platelet count) indicate severe or worsening coagulopathy, the risk of continuing the infusion should be weighed against the expected benefit

- *Xigris* should not be used during pregnancy or lactation unless clearly necessary

See appendix H

Organ failure

Renal: no dose adjustments required
Hepatic: no dose adjustments required

ENOXIMONE

Enoximone is a selective phosphodiesterase III inhibitor resulting in ↑ CO, and ↓PCWP and SVR, without significant ↑ in HR and myocardial oxygen consumption. It has a long half-life and haemodynamic effects can persist for 8–10 h after the drug is stopped.

Uses
Severe congestive cardiac failure
Low cardiac output states (± dobutamine)

Contraindications
Severe aortic or pulmonary stenosis (exaggerated hypotension)
HOCM (exaggerated hypotension)

Administration
- IV infusion: 0.5–1.0 mg/kg, then 5–20 mcg/kg/min maintenance

Requires direct arterial BP monitoring
Adjustment of the infusion rate should be made according to haemodynamic response
Total dose in 24 h should not >24 mg/kg
Available in 20-ml ampoules containing 100 mg enoximone (5 mg/ml)
Dilute this 20 ml solution with 20 ml 0.9% saline giving a solution containing enoximone 2.5 mg/ml

How not to use enoximone
5% Dextrose or contact with glass may result in crystal formation
Do not dilute with very alkaline solution (incompatible with all catecholamines in solution)

Adverse effects
Hypotension
Arrhythmias

Cautions
In septic shock enoximone can cause prolonged hypotension

Organ failure
Renal: reduce dose

Renal replacement therapy
No further dose modification is required during renal replacement therapy

EPOETIN

E

Epoetin (recombinant human erythropoetin) is available as epoetin alfa and beta. Both are similar in clinical efficacy and can be used inter-changeably.

Uses
Anaemia associated with erythropoetin deficiency in chronic renal failure
Severe anaemia due to blood loss in Jehovah's witness (unlicensed)

Contraindications
Uncontrolled hypertension
Anaemia due to iron, folic acid or vitamin B_{12} deficiency

Administration
- Chronic renal failure

Aim to increase haemoglobin concentration at rate not $>2 g/100 ml$ per month to stable level of $10-12 g/100 ml$
SC (maximum 1 ml per injection site) or IV given over 3–5 min
Initially 50 units/kg three times weekly increased according to response in steps of 25 units/kg at intervals of 4 weeks
Maintenance dose (when haemoglobin $10-12 g/100 ml$) 50–300 units/kg weekly in 2–3 divided doses

- Severe anaemia due to blood loss in Jehovah's witness

150–300 units/kg daily SC until desired haemoglobin reached
Supplementary iron (e.g. ferrous sulphate 200 mg PO) and O_2 is mandatory
Monitor:
BP, haemoglobin, serum ferritin, platelet, and electrolytes

How not to use epoetin
Avoid contact of reconstituted injection with glass; use only plastic materials

Adverse effects
Dose-dependent increase in BP and platelet count
Flu-like symptoms (reduced if IV given over 5 min)
Shunt thrombosis
Hyperkalaemia
Increase in plasma urea, creatinine and phosphate
Convulsions
Skin reactions
Palpebral oedema
Myocardial infarction
Anaphylaxis

Cautions
Hypertension (stop if uncontrolled)
Ischaemic vascular disease
Thrombocytosis (monitor platelet count for first 8 weeks)
Epilepsy
Malignant disease
Chronic liver disease

EPOPROSTENOL (Flolan)

Epoprostenol has a half-life of only 3 min and must be given by continuous IV infusion. It is a potent vasodilator and therefore its side-effects includes flushing, headaches and hypotension. Epoprostenol may be used instead of or as well as heparin during haemofiltration to inhibit platelet aggregation. The dose is dictated by clinical need and filter life (ideally at least 2–3 days).

Uses
Haemofiltration (unlicensed)
ARDS (unlicensed)

Administration
• Haemofiltration

IV infusion: 2–10 ng/kg/min, start 1 h before haemofiltration
Available in vials containing 500 mcg epoprostenol. Stored in fridge
Reconstitute the powder with the 50 ml diluent provided (concentration 10 000 ng/ml). Take 10 ml this reconstituted solution and further dilute with 40 ml 0.9% saline into a 50 ml syringe (concentration 2000 ng/ml)

Dosage chart (ml/h)

Weight (kg)	Dose (ng/kg/min)			
	2	3	4	5
50	3.0	4.5	6.0	7.5
60	3.6	5.4	7.2	9.0
70	4.2	6.3	8.4	10.5
80	4.8	7.2	9.6	12.0
90	5.4	8.1	10.8	13.5
100	6.0	9.0	12.0	15.0

• ARDS

Nebulized: 4 ml/h of the reconstituted powder (500 mcg epoprostenol reconstituted with the 50 ml diluent provided) into ventilator circuit

Adverse effects
Flushing
Headaches
Hypotension
Bradycardia

E

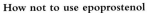

How not to use epoprostenol

For haemofiltration, epoprostenol is given by IV infusion into the patient and not into the extracorporeal circuit

Cautions

Epoprostenol may potentiate heparin

*reconstitute
with 20mls water WFI → then NaCl
if IV*

ERYTHROMYCIN

Erythromycin has an antibacterial spectrum similar but not identical to that of penicillin; it is thus an alternative in penicillin-allergic patients. Resistance rates in Gram +ve organisms limit its use for severe soft tissue infections. Erythromycin has also been used as a prokinetic in gastric stasis and in aiding the passage of fine-bore feeding tube beyond the pylorus. Erythromycin is an agonist at motilin receptors. Motilin is a peptide secreted in the small intestine, which induces GI contractions, so increasing gut motility. Use as a prokinetic may increase patient colonisation with resistant bacterial species including MRSA.

Uses
Alternative to penicillin
Community acquired pneumonia, particularly caused by atypical organisms
Infective exacerbations of COPD
Legionnaire's disease
Pharyngeal and sinus infections
As a prokinetic (unlicensed)

Administration
* IV infusion: 0.5–1.0 g 6 hourly
Reconstitute with 20 ml WFI, shake well, then further dilute in 250 ml 0.9% saline, given over 1 h
In severe renal impairment: maximum 1.5 g daily
* As a prokinetic: 125 mg 6 hourly PO/NG   *– bowel movement*

How not to use erythromycin
IV bolus is not recommended
No other diluent (apart from WFI) should be used for the initial reconstitution
Do not use concurrently with astemizole or terfenadine

Adverse effects
Gastrointestinal intolerance
Hypersensitivity reactions
Reversible hearing loss with large doses
Cholestatic jaundice if given >14 days
Prolongation of QT interval

Cautions
↑ Plasma levels of alfentanil, midazolam and theophylline
Severe renal impairment (ototoxicity)
Hepatic disease

Organ failure
Renal: reduce dose

Renal replacement therapy
No further dose modification is required during renal replacement therapy

ie 250mg in 100 ml NaCl in 30 mins

beta-Blocker

ESMOLOL (Brevibloc)

Esmolol is a relatively cardioselective b-blocker with a rapid onset and a very short duration of action. Esmolol is metabolized by esterases in the red blood cells and the elimination half-life is about 9 min. It is used IV for the short-term treatment of supraventricular arrhythmias, sinus tachycardia, or hypertension and is particularly useful in the peri-operative period.

Uses
AF
Atrial flutter
Sinus tachycardia
Hypertension

Contraindications
Unstable asthma
Severe bradycardia
Sick sinus syndrome
Second- or third-degree AV block
Uncontrolled heart failure
Hypotension

Administration
- IV bolus: 80 mg loading bolus over 15–30 s, followed by IV infusion
- IV infusion: 50–200 mcg/kg/min (210–840 or 21–84 ml/h in a 70 kg individual)

Available in 10-ml vial containing 100 mg esmolol (10 mg/ml) to be used undiluted and 10 ml ampoule containing 2.5 g esmolol (250 mg/ml) requiring dilution to 10 mg/ml solution. Dilute 5 g (two ampoules) in 500 ml 0.9% saline or 5% dextrose (10 mg/ml)

How not to use esmolol
Not compatible with sodium bicarbonate
Esmolol 2.5 g ampoules must be diluted before infusion

Cautions
Asthma

Adverse effects
Bradycardia
Heart failure
Hypotension
These side-effects should resolve within 30 min of discontinuing infusion

FENTANYL

Fentanyl is 100 times as potent as morphine. Its onset of action is within 1–2 min after IV injection and a peak effect within 4–5 min. Duration of action after a single bolus is 20 min. The context sensitive half-life following IV infusion is prolonged because of its large volume of distribution.

Uses
Analgesia

Contraindications
Airway obstruction

Administration
• For sedation

IV infusion: 1–5 microgram/kg/h

• During anaesthesia

IV bolus:

• 1–3 microgram/kg with spontaneous ventilation
• 5–10 microgram/kg with IPPV
• 7–10 microgram/kg to obtund pressor response of laryngoscopy
• Up to 100 microgram/kg for cardiac surgery

How not to use fentanyl
In combination with an opioid partial agonist, e.g. buprenorphine (antagonizes opioid effects)

Adverse effects
Respiratory depression and apnoea
Bradycardia and hypotension
Nausea and vomiting
Delayed gastric emptying
Reduce intestinal mobility
Biliary spasm
Constipation
Urinary retention
Chest wall rigidity (may interfere with ventilation)
Muscular rigidity and hypotension more common after high dosage

Cautions

Enhanced sedation and respiratory depression from interaction with:

- benzodiazepines
- antidepressants
- anti-psychotics

Head injury and neurosurgical patients (may exacerbate – ICP as a result of – $PaCO_2$)

Organ failure

Respiratory: – respiratory depression
Hepatic: enhanced and prolonged sedative effect

FLUCLOXACILLIN

A derivative of the basic penicillin structure which has stability to the staphylococcal penicillinase found in most *Staphylococcus aureus* isolates. Generally less active than benzylpenicillin against other Gram +ve organisms. Strains which express resistance are designated methicillin resistant and are known as MRSAs.

Uses
Infections due to penicillinase-producing staphylococci (except MRSA):

- cellulitis
- wound infection
- endocarditis
- adjunct in pneumonia
- osteomyelitis
- septic arthritis

Contraindications
Penicillin hypersensitivity

Administration
IV: 0.25–2 g 6 hourly, depending on the severity of infection. For endo-carditis (in combination with another antibiotic), 2 g 6 hourly, increasing to 2 g 4 hourly if over 85 kg.

Infection	Dose (g)	Interval (h)
Mild – moderate	0.25–0.5	6
Moderate – serious	1–2	6
Life-threatening	2	6

Reconstitute with 20 ml WFI, given over 3–5 min

How not to use flucloxacillin
Not for intrathecal use (encephlopathy)
Do not mix in the same syringe with an aminoglycoside (efficacy of aminoglycoside reduced)

F

Adverse effects
Hypersensitivity
Haemolytic anaemia
Transient neutropenia and thrombocytopenia
Cholestatic jaundice and hepatitis
– ↑ risk with treatment >2 weeks and increasing age
– may occur up to several weeks after stopping treatment

Cautions
Liver failure (worsening of LFTs)

Organ failure
Renal: reduce dose
Hepatic: avoid

Renal replacement therapy
No further dose modification is required during renal replacement therapy

FLUCONAZOLE

Antifungal active against *Candida albicans, Candida tropicalis, Candida parapsilosis* and cryptococcus. Variable activity against *Candida glabrata* and poor activity for *Candida krusei*. It is rapidly and completely absorbed orally. Oral and IV therapy equally effective; IV for patients unable to take orally. Widely distributed in tissues and fluids. Excreted unchanged in urine.

Uses
Local or systemic candidiasis
Cryptococcal infections – usually follow on therapy after amphotericin

Administration
* Oropharyngeal candidiasis
Orally: 50–100 mg daily for 7–14 days
* Oesophageal candidiasis or candiduria
Orally: 50–100 mg daily for 14–30 days
* Systemic candidiasis or cryptococcal infections
IV infusion: 400 mg initially, then 200–400 mg daily, consider higher doses for less susceptible Candida isolates
Do not give at rate >200 mg/hr
Continued according to response (at least 6–8 weeks for cryptococcal meningitis; often longer)
In renal impairment:
Normal doses on days 1 and 2, then:

CC (ml/min)	Dosage interval/daily dose
>40	24 h (normal dosage regime)
21-40	48 h or half normal daily dose
10-20	72 h or one-third normal daily dose

How not to use fluconazole
Avoid concurrent use with astemizole or terfenadine (arrhythmias)

Adverse effects
Rash
Pruritis
Nausea, vomiting, diarrhoea
Raised liver enzymes
Hypersensitivity

Cautions
Renal/hepatic impairment
May increase concentrations of cyclosporin, phenytoin

F

Organ failure
Renal: reduce dose

Renal replacement therapy
Removed by HD / HF / PD but significant only for high clearance technique. For high clearance technique consider increased dose over that for normal renal function, halve dose if low clearance. For intermittent renal therapy give half dose after each treatment.

FLUMAZENIL

A competitive antagonist at the benzodiazepine receptor. It has a short duration of action (20 min).

Uses
To facilitate weaning from ventilation in patients sedated with benzodiazepine
In the management of benzodiazepine overdose
As a diagnostic test for the cause of prolonged sedation

Contraindications
Tricyclic antidepressant and mixed-drug overdose (fits)
Patients on long-term benzodiazepine therapy (withdrawal)
Epileptic patients on benzodiazepines (fits)
Patients with raised ICP (further increase in ICP)

Administration
- IV bolus: 200 microgram, repeat at 1-min intervals until desired response, up to a total dose of 2 mg

If resedation occurs, repeat dose every 20 min

How not to use flumazenil
Ensure effects of neuromuscular blockade reversed before using flumazenil

Adverse effects
Dizziness
Agitation
Arrhythmias
Hypertension
Epileptic fits

Cautions
Resedation – requires prolonged monitoring if long-acting benzodiazepines have been taken

Organ failure
Hepatic: reduced elimination

FUROSEMIDE

A widely used loop diuretic.

Uses
Acute oliguric renal failure – may convert acute oliguric to non-oliguric renal failure. Other measures must be taken to ensure adequate circulating blood volume and renal perfusion pressure
Pulmonary oedema – secondary to acute left ventricular failure
Oedema – associated with congestive cardiac failure, hepatic failure and renal disease

Contraindications
Oliguria secondary to hypovolaemia

Administration
- IV bolus: 10–40 mg over 3–5 min
- IV infusion: 2–10 mg/h

For high-dose parenteral therapy (up to 1000 mg/day), dilute in 250–500 ml 0.9% saline given at a rate not >240 mg/h

How not to use furosemide
Dextrose containing fluid is not recommended as a diluent (infusion pH >5.5, otherwise may precipitate)
Do not give at >240 mg/h (transient deafness)

Adverse effects
Hyponatraemia, hypokalaemia, hypomagnesaemia
Hyperuricaemia, hyperglycaemia
Ototoxicity
Nephrotoxicity
Pancreatitis

Cautions
Amphotericin (increased risk of hypokalaemia)
Aminoglycosides (increased nephrotoxicity and ototoxicity)
Digoxin toxicity (due to hypokalaemia)

Organ failure
Renal: may need to increase dose for effect

Renal replacement therapy
No further dose modification is required during renal replacement therapy

GANCICLOVIR (Cymevene)

G

Ganciclovir is related to aciclovir but is more active against cytomegalovirus (CMV). It is also more toxic. It causes profound myelo-suppression when given with zidovudine; the two should not be given together particularly during initial ganciclovir therapy.

Uses
CMV infections in immunocompromised patients
Prevention of CMV infection during immunosuppression following organ transplantation

Contraindications
Hypersensitivity to ganciclovir and aciclovir
Abnormally low neutrophil counts

Administration
- IV infusion: 5 mg/kg 12 hourly, given over 1 h through filter provided

Reconstitute the 500 mg powder with 10 ml WFI, then dilute with 50–100 ml 0.9% saline or 5% dextrose
Wear polythene gloves and safety glasses when preparing solution
Duration of treatment: 7–14 days for prevention and 14–21 days for treatment
Ensure adequate hydration
Monitor: FBC
              U&E
              LFT
In renal impairment:

Serum creatinine (μmol/l)	Dose (mg/kg)	Interval (h)
<124	5.0	12
125–225	2.5	12
226–398	2.5	24
>398	1.25	24

Adverse effects
Leucopenia
Thrombocytopenia
Anaemia
Fever
Rash
Abnormal LFT

G

Cautions
History of cytopenia, low platelet count
Concurrent use of myelosuppressants
Renal impairment

Renal replacement therapy
The major route of clearance of ganciclovir is by glomerular filtration of the unchanged drug. Removed by HD and HF similar to urea clearance, only likely to be significant for high clearance systems. Dose on the basis of the achieved serum creatinine (see table). For intermittent renal therapy give dose after treatment. Clearance by PD not likely to achieve clinical significance

GENTAMICIN

G

This is the aminoglycoside most commonly used in the UK. It is effective against Gram –ve organisms such as *E. coli*, *Klebsiella* spp., *Proteus* spp., *Serratia* spp and *Pseudomonas aeruginosa*. It is also active against *Staphylococcus aureus*. It is inactive against anaerobes and has poor activity against all streptococci including *Strep. pyogenes* and *Strep. pneumoniae*, and *Enterococus* spp. When given in combination with a penicillin, excellent synergy is achieved against most strains of s*treptococci* and *enterococci*. When used for the 'blind' therapy of undiagnosed serious infections it is usually given with a penicillin and metronidazole, if indicated (e.g. abdominal sepsis).

It is not appreciably absorbed orally and is renally excreted unchanged. In renal impairment the half-life is prolonged. Most side-effects are related to sustained high trough concentrations. Efficacy, on the other hand, is related to peak concentrations that are well in excess of the minimum inhibitory concentration of the infecting organism. Plasma concentration monitoring is essential.

High dose single daily dosing of aminoglycosides has become more popular recently. It ensures that target peak concentrations are achieved in all patients and may also be less nephrotoxic. It also makes monitoring of gentamicin levels easier.

Uses
- Sepsis of unknown origin (with a penicillin and/or metronidazole)
- Intra-abdominal infections (with a penicillin and metronidazole)
- Acute pyelonephritis (with ampicillin)
- Infective endocarditis (with a penicillin)
- Hospital acquired pneumonia (with a 3rd generation cephalosporin)
- Severe infections due to *P. aeruginosa* (with ceftazidime or piperacillin/tazobactam)
- Enterococcal infections (with a penicillin)
- Febrile neutropenia (with ceftazidime or piperacillin/tazobactam)

Contraindications
Pregnancy
Myasthenia gravis

G

Administration

• Rapid IV bolus: 1.5 mg/kg IV 8 hourly

In renal impairment:

CC (ml/min)	Dose (mg/kg)	Interval (h)
20–50	1.5	12–24
10–20	1.0–1.5	12–24
<10	1.0	24–48

Monitor plasma level (p. 193): adjust dose/interval accordingly

• High dose single daily dosing protocol

IV infusion: 7 mg/kg in 50 ml 5% dextrose or 0.9% saline, given over 1 hour. For obese patients lean body weight should be used (see Appendix D). The interval is then decided after referring to the Hartford nomogram (developed and validated by DP Nicolau et al., Division of infectious Diseases, Hartford Hospital, Hartford, Connecticut, USA). A blood level is taken after the first dose to determine subsequent dosing interval. Nomograms have also been developed for 5 mg/kg.

Monitoring: Take a single blood sample at any time 6–14 hr after the **start** of an IV infusion. It is essential that the **exact** time is recorded accurately.

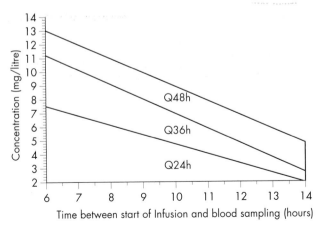

Evaluate on the nomogram. If the level lies in the area designated Q24, Q36 or Q48, the interval should be every 24, 36 or 48 hourly respectively. Frequency of repeat levels depends on underlying renal function.

If the point is on the line, choose the longer interval. If the dosing interval is greater than 48 hours, an alternative artibiotic should be used. Single daily dosing should not be used for children, pregnant women, burns patients, infective endocarditis and patients with significant pre-existing renal impairment. It should be used with caution in very septic patients with incipient renal failure.

How not to use gentamicin
Do not mix in a syringe with penicillins and cephalosporins (amino-glycosides inactivated)

Adverse effects
Nephrotoxicity – ↑ risk with amphotericin, bumetanide, furosemide, vancomycin and lithium
Ototoxicity – ↑ risk with pre-existing renal insufficiency, elderly, bumetanide, furosemide
Prolonged neuromuscular blockade – may be clinically significant in patients being weaned from mechanical ventilation

Cautions
Renal impairment (reduce dose)
Concurrent use of:

• amphotericin – ↑ nephrotoxicity

• bumetanide, frusemide – ↑ ototoxicity

• neuromuscular blockers – prolonged muscle weakness

Organ failure
Renal: increased plasma concentration – ↑ ototoxicity and nephrotoxicity

Renal replacement therapy
Removed by HD/HF/PD. Levels must be monitored, and dose and interval adjusted accordingly. Dose according to achieved creatinine clearance. For intermittent therapy give after treatment.

GENTAMICIN

GLUTAMINE

Glutamine is primarily synthesized in skeletal muscle and is the most abundant amino acid. It is a major metabolic fuel for the enterocytes in the gut mucosa. Glutamine is also required for lymphocyte and macrophage function, and is a precursor for nucleotide synthesis. Glutathione is a product of glutamine metabolism, and has an important role as an antioxidant. Although not regarded as an essential amino acid, it becomes conditionally essential in catabolic states. Surgery, trauma or sepsis decreases plasma concentrations. Some studies have shown that glutamine supplemented enteral feeds improve nitrogen balance, reduce infections and length of hospital stay. This may, at least in part, be explained by the reduced bacterial translocation. However, none of these studies have shown improved survival when compared with standard feeds (p. 219).

Uses
Immunonutrition – to maintain gut integrity and prevent bacterial translocation during critical illness

Administration
Orally: 5 g 6 hourly
Dissolve the 5 g sachet in 20 ml WFI

Cautions
Phenylketonuria (contains aspartame)

GLYCEROL SUPPOSITORY

Glycerol suppositories act as a rectal stimulant by virtue of the mildly irritant action of glycerol.

Uses
Constipation

Contraindications
Intestinal obstruction

Administration
PR: 4 g suppository moistened with water before insertion

How not to use glycerol suppository
Not for prolonged use

Adverse effects
Abdominal discomfort

Cautions
Prolonged use (atonic colon and hypokalaemia)

HALOPERIDOL

A butyrophenone with longer duration of action than droperidol. It has anti-emetic and neuroleptic effects with minimal cardiovascular and respiratory effects. It is a mild α-blocker and may cause hypotension in the presence of hypovolaemia.

Uses
Acute agitation

Contraindications
Agitation caused by hypoxia, hypoglycaemia or a full bladder
Parkinson's disease

Administration
- IV bolus: 2.5–5 mg
- IM: 5–10 mg

5mg vial make up to 10mls (1mg in 2mls)

Up to every 4–8 h

How not to use haloperidol
Hypotension resulting from haloperidol should not be treated with adrenaline as a further decrease in BP may result

Adverse effects
Extra-pyramidal movements
Neuroleptic malignant syndrome (treat with dantrolene)

Cautions
Concurrent use of other CNS depressants (enhanced sedation)

Organ failure
CNS: sedative effects increased
Hepatic: can precipitate coma
Renal: increased cerebral sensitivity

Renal replacement therapy
No further dose modification is required during renal replacement therapy

HEPARIN

Uses
Prophylaxis of DVT and PE
Treatment of DVT and PE
Extracorporeal circuits

Contraindications
Haemophilia and other haemorrhagic disorders
Peptic ulcer
Cerebral haemorrhage
Severe hypertension
Severe liver disease (including oesophageal varices)
Severe renal failure
Thrombocytopenia
Hypersensitivity to heparin

Administration
• Prophylaxis of DVT and PE

SC: 5000 units 8–12 hourly until patient is ambulant

• Treatment of DVT and PE

IV: Loading dose of 5000 units followed by continuous infusion of 1000–2000 units/h
24 000 units heparin made up to 48 ml with 0.9% saline (5000 units/ml). Check APTT 6 h after loading dose and adjust rate to keep APTT between 1.5 and 2.5 times normal
Start oral warfarin as soon as possible

• Haemofiltration

1000 units to run through the system. Then a bolus of 1500–3000 units injected into the pre-filter port, followed by 5–10 units/kg/h infused into the pre-filter port
Dose is dictated by clinical need and filter life (ideally at least 2–3 days)

Adverse effects
Haemorrhage
Skin necrosis
Thrombocytopenia
Hypersensitivity
Osteoporosis after prolonged use

Cautions
Hepatic and renal impairment (avoid if severe)

HYDRALAZINE (Apresoline)

Hydralazine lowers the BP by reducing arterial resistance through a direct relaxation of arteriolar smooth muscle. This effect is limited by reflex tachycardia and so it is best combined with a β-blocker. Metabolism occurs by hepatic acetylation, the rate of which is genetically determined. Fast acetylators show a reduced therapeutic effect until the enzyme system is saturated.

Uses
All grades of hypertension
Pre-eclampsia

Contraindications
Systemic lupus erythematosus
Dissecting aortic aneurysm
Right ventricular failure due to pulmonary hypertension (cor pulmonale)
Severe tachycardia and heart failure with a high cardiac output state, e.g. thyrotoxicosis
Severe aortic outflow obstruction (aortic stenosis, mitral stenosis, constrictive pericarditis)

Administration
• IV bolus: 10–20 mg over 3–5 min

Reconstitute the ampoule containing 20 mg powder with 1 ml WFI, further dilute with 10 ml 0.9% saline, give over 3–5 min
Expect to see response after 20 min
Repeat after 20–30 min as necessary

• IV infusion: 2–15 mg/h

Reconstitute three ampoules (60 mg) of hydralazine with 1 ml WFI each. Make up to 60 ml with 0.9% saline (1 mg/ml)
Give at a rate between 2 and 15 mg/h depending on the BP and pulse
Rapid acetylators may require higher doses

How not to use hydralazine
Do not dilute in fluids containing dextrose (glucose causes breakdown of hydralazine)

Adverse effects
Headache
Tachycardia
Hypotension
Myocardial ischaemia
Sodium and fluid retention, producing oedema and reduced urinary volume (prevented by concomitant use of a diuretic)
Lupus erythematosus (commoner if slow acetylator status, women, and if treatment >6 months at doses >100 mg daily)

Cautions

Cerebrovascular disease

Cardiac disease (angina, immediately post-MI)

Use with other antihypertensives and nitrate drugs may produce additive hypotensive effects

Organ failure

Hepatic: prolonged effect

Renal: increased hypotensive effect (start with small dose)

HYDROCORTISONE

In the critically ill patient, adrenocortical insufficiency should be considered when an inappropriate amount of inotropic support is required. Baseline cortisol levels and short synacthen test do not predict response to steroid. In patients who demonstrate a normal short synacthen test, but yet show a dramatic response to steroid, it is possible that the abnormality lies in altered receptor function or glucocorticoid resistance rather than abnormality of the adrenal axis. Baseline cortisol levels and short synacthen test are worthwhile to assess hypothalamic–pituitary–adrenal axis dysfunction versus steroid unresponsiveness.

Available as the sodium succinate or the phosphate ester

Uses
Adrenal insufficiency (primary or secondary)
Severe bronchospasm
Hypersensitivity reactions (p. 200)
Fibroproliferative phase of ARDS (unlicensed)
Adjunct in *Pneumocystis carinii* pneumonia (see co-trimoxazole and pentamidine)

Contraindications
Systemic infection (unless specific anti-microbial therapy given)

Administration
• Adrenal insufficiency

Major surgery or stress: IV 100–500 mg 6–8 hourly
Minor surgery: IV 50 mg 8–12 hourly
Reduce by 25% per day until normal oral steroids resumed or maintained on 20 mg in the morning and 10 mg in the evening IV

• Prolonged vasopressor dependent shock

Initial dose 50 mg IV bolus, followed by infusion of 10 mg/h for up to 48 h

• Fibroproliferative phase of ARDS

IV infusion: 100–200 mg 6 hourly for up to 3 days, then dose reduced gradually

• Adjunct in *Pneumocystis carinii* pneumonia (see co-trimoxazole and pentamidine)

IV: 100 mg 6 hourly for 5 days, then dose reduced to complete 21 days of treatment
The steroid should be started at the same time as the co-trimoxazole or pentamidine and should be withdrawn before the antibiotic treatment is complete.
Reconstitute 100 mg powder with 2 ml WFI. Further dilute 200 mg and made up to 40 ml with 0.9% saline or 5% dextrose (5 mg/ml)

How not to use hydrocortisone
Do not stop abruptly (adrenocortical insufficiency)

Adverse effects
Perineal irritation may follow IV administration of the phosphate ester
Prolonged use may also lead to the following problems:

- Increased susceptibility to infections
- Impaired wound healing
- Peptic ulceration
- Muscle weakness (proximal myopathy)
- Osteoporosis
- Hyperglycaemia

Cautions
Diabetes mellitus
Concurrent use of NSAID (increased risk of GI bleeding)

IMIPENEM + CILASTATIN (Primaxin)

Imipenem is given in combination with cilastatin, a specific inhibitor of the renal enzyme dehydropeptidase-1 that inactivates imipenem. Imipenem has an extremely wide spectrum of activity, including most aerobic and anaerobic Gram −ve, including those expressing extended spectrum beta-lactamases, and Gram +ve bacteria (but not MRSA). It has no activity against *Stenotrophomonas maltophilia* which emerges in some patients treated with imipenem. Acquired resistance is relatively common in *P. aeruginosa* and is starting to emerge in some of the Enterobacteriaceae including *Enterobacter* spp., *Citrobacter* spp. and the proteus group.

Uses
- Mixed aerobic/anaerobic infections
- Presumptive therapy prior to availability of sensitivities for a wide range of severe infections
- Febrile neutropenia

Contraindications
CNS infections (neurotoxicity)
Meningitis (neurotoxicity)

Administration
- IV infusion: 0.5–1 g 6–8 hourly depending on severity of infection

Dilute with 0.9% saline or 5% dextrose to a concentration of 5 mg/ml
500 mg: add 100 ml diluent, infuse over 30 min
1 g: add 200 ml diluent, infuse over 60 min
Unstable at room temperature following reconstitution – use immediately

In renal impairment:

CC (ml/min)	Dose (g)	Interval (h)
20–50	0.5	6–8
10–20	0.5	8–12
<10	0.5	12–24

How not to use imipenem
Not compatible with diluents containing lactate

Adverse effects
Hypersensitivity reactions
Blood disorders
Positive Coombs' test
↑ Liver function tests, serum creatinine and blood urea
Myoclonic activity
Convulsions (high doses or renal impairment)

Cautions
Hypersensitivity to penicillins and cephalosporins
Renal impairment
Elderly

Organ failure
Renal: reduce dose

Renal replacement therapy
No further dose modification is required during renal replacement therapy

IMMUNOGLOBULINS

Human normal immunoglobulin is prepared by cold alcohol fractionation of pooled plasma from over 1000 donations. Individual donor units of plasma are screened for hepatitis B surface antigen (HBsAg) and for the presence of antibodies to human immunodeficiency virus type 1 (HIV-1), HIV-2, or hepatitis C virus (HCV) which, combined with careful donor selection, minimises the risk of viral transmission. In addition, the testing for HBsAg, HIV-1, HIV-2 and HCV antibodies is repeated on the plasma pools.

Uses
Guillain-Barré syndrome
Weakness during exacerbations in Myasthenia Gravis (unlicensed)

Contraindications
Patients with known class specific antibody to IgA (risk of anaphylactoid reactions)

Administration
- For Guillain Barré syndrome and myasthenia gravis

IV infusion: 0.4 g/kg IV daily for 5 consecutive days. Repeat at 4 week intervals if necessary.
Patient treated for the first time: give at rate of 30 ml/h, if no adverse effect occur within 15 min, increase rate to maximum of 150 ml/h.
Subsequent infusions: give at rate of 100 ml/h.
Once reconstituted, avoid shaking the bottle (risk of foaming). The solution should be used only if it is clear, and given without delay.

How not to use immunoglobulins
Should not be mixed with any other drug and should always be given through a separate infusion line.
Live virus vaccines (except yellow fever) should be given at least 3 weeks before or 3 months after an injection of normal immunoglobulin.

Adverse effects
Chills
Fever
Transient ↑ serum creatinine
Anaphylaxis (rare)

INSULIN

Insulin plays a key role in the regulation of carbohydrate, fat and protein metabolism. Hyperglycaemia and insulin resistance are common in critically ill patients even if they have not previously had diabetes. A recent study (Van den Berghe G, et al. *New England Journal of Medicine* 2001; 345: 1349–67) has shown that tight control of blood glucose levels (between 4.4 and 6.1 mmol/L) reduces mortality among intensive care patients even in patients who do not previously have diabetes. The incidence of complications such as septicaemia, acute renal failure and critical illness polyneuropathy may also be reduced.

Uses
• Hyperglycaemia
• Emergency treatment of hyperkalaemia (p. 201)

Administration
• Hyperglycaemia

Soluble insulin (e.g. Actrapid) 50 units made up to 50 ml with 0.9% saline
Adjust rate according to the sliding scale below
Insulin sliding scale

Blood sugar (mmol/l)	Rate (ml/h)
<3.5	0
3.6–5.5	1
5.6–7.0	2
7.1–9.0	3
9.1–11.0	4
11.1–17.0	5
>17.0	6

The energy and carbohydrate intake must be adequate; this may be in the form of entereal or parenteral feeding, or IV infusion of 10% dextrose containing 10–40 mmol/l KCl running at a constant rate appropriate to the patient's fluid requirements (85–125 ml/h). The blood glucose concentration should be maintained between 4 and 10 mmol/l.
Monitor:
Blood glucose 2 hourly until stable then 4 hourly
Serum potassium 12 hourly

How not to use insulin
SC administration not recommended for fine control
Adsorption of insulin occurs with PVC bags (use polypropylene syringes)

Adverse effects
Hypoglycaemia

Cautions
Insulin resistance may occur in patients with high levels of IgG antibodies to insulin, obesity, acanthosis nigricans and insulin receptor defects.

IPRATROPIUM

An antimuscarinic bronchodilator traditionally regarded as more effective in relieving bronchoconstriction associated with COPD.

Uses
Reverse bronchospasm, particularly in COPD

Administration
- Nebulizer: 250–500 microgram up to 6 hourly, undiluted (if prolonged delivery time desirable then dilute with 0.9% saline only)

For patients with chronic bronchitis and hypercapnia, oxygen in high concentration can be dangerous, and nebulizers should be driven by air

How not to use ipratropium
For nebulizer: do not dilute in anything other than 0.9% saline (hypotonic solution may cause bronchospasm)

Adverse effects
Dry mouth
Tachycardia
Paradoxical bronchospasm (stop giving if suspected)
Acute angle closure glaucoma (avoid escape from mask to patient's eyes)

Cautions
Prostatic hypertrophy – urinary retention (unless patient's bladder catheterized)

ISOPRENALINE

Isoprenaline is a β_1 and β_2 adrenoceptor agonist causing: ↑ HR, ↑ automaticity, ↑ contractility, ↓ diastolic BP, ↑ systolic BP, ↑ myocardial oxygen demand and bronchodilation. It has a half-life of <5 min.

Uses
Complete heart block, while getting temporary pacing established

Contraindications
Tachyarrhythmias
Heartblock caused by digoxin

Administration
• IV infusion: up to 20 microgram/min

4 mg made up to 50 ml 5% dextrose (80 microgram/ml)

Dose (microgram/min)	Infusion rate (ml/h)
1	0.75
2	1.5
4	3
10	7.5
20	15

How not to use isoprenaline
Do not use 0.9% saline as a diluent

Adverse effects
Tachycardia
Arrhythmias
Angina
Hypotension

Cautions
Risk of arrhythmias with concurrent use of other sympathomimetics and volatile anaesthetics

LABETALOL (Trandate)

Labetalol is a combined α- and β-adrenoceptor antagonist. The proportion of β-blockade to α-blockade when given orally is 3:1, and 7:1 when given IV. It lowers the blood pressure by blocking α-adrenoceptors in arterioles and thereby reducing the peripheral resistance. Concurrent β-blockade protects the heart from reflex sympathetic drive normally induced by peripheral vasodilatation.

Uses
All grades of hypertension, particularly useful when there is tachycardia
Pre-eclampsia

Contraindications
Asthma (worsens)
Cardiogenic shock (further myocardial depression)
Second- or third-degree heart block

Administration
- Orally: 100–800 mg 12 hourly

- IV bolus: 10–20 mg over 2 min, repeat with 40 mg at 10 min intervals as necessary, up to 300 mg in 24 h

Maximum effect usually occurs within 5 min and the duration of action is usually 6 h

- IV Infusion: 20–160 mg/h

Rate: 4–32 ml/h (20–160 mg/h), adjust rate until satisfactory ≈ BP obtained
Available in 20 ml ampoules containing 100 mg labetalol (5 mg/ml)
Draw up three ampoules (60 ml) into a 50 ml syringe

How not to use labetalol
Incompatible with sodium bicarbonate

Adverse effects
Postural hypotension
Bradycardia
Heart failure

Cautions
Rare reports of severe hepatocellular damage (usually reversible)
Presence of labetalol metabolites in urine may result in false positive test for phaeochromocytoma

Organ failure
Hepatic: reduce dose

LACTULOSE

Lactulose is a semi-synthetic disaccharide that is not absorbed from the GI tract. It produces an osmotic diarrhoea of low faecal pH, and discourages the proliferation of ammonia-producing organisms.

Uses
Constipation
Hepatic encephalopathy

Contraindications
Intestinal obstruction
Galactosaemia

Administration
• Constipation

Orally: 15 ml 12 hourly, gradually reduced according to patient's needs
May take up to 48 h to act

• Hepatic encephalopathy

Orally: 30–50 ml 8 hourly, subsequently adjusted to produce 2–3 soft stools daily

Adverse effects
Flatulence
Abdominal discomfort

LIDOCAINE

This anti-arrhythmic agent suppresses automaticity of conduction and spontaneous depolarization of the ventricles during diastole. Clearance is related to both hepatic blood flow and hepatic function; it will be prolonged in liver disease, cardiac failure and the elderly. The effects after the initial bolus dose last about 20 min. An IV infusion is needed to maintain the anti-arrhythmic effect.

Uses
Prevention of ventricular ectopic beats, VT and VF after MI

Contraindications
It is no longer the first-line drug in pulseless VT or VF during cardiac arrest
Hypersensitivity to amide-type local anaesthetics (rare)
Heart block (risk of asystole)

Administration
• Loading dose:

1.5 mg/kg IV over 2 min, repeat after 5 min to a total dose of 3 mg/kg if necessary. Reduce dose in the elderly

• Maintenance dose:

4 mg/min for 1st h
2 mg/min for 2nd h
1 mg/min thereafter
Reduce infusion rates in patients with hepatic impairment, cardiac failure and in the elderly
Undiluted 40 ml 2 % solution (800 mg)
4 mg/min = 12 ml/h
2 mg/min = 6 ml/h
1 mg/min = 3 ml/h
Continuous ECG and BP monitoring

How not to use lidocaine
Do not give by rapid IV bolus (should not be given at >50 mg/min)

Adverse effects
Paraesthesia, muscle twitching, tinnitus
Anxiety, drowsiness, confusion, convulsions
Hypotension, bradycardia, asystole

Cautions
Elderly (reduced volume of distribution, reduce dose by 50%)
Hepatic impairment
Cardiac failure
Other class 1 anti-arrhythmics, e.g. phenytoin, may increase risk of toxicity

Organ failure
Cardiac: reduce dose
Hepatic: reduce dose

LINEZOLID (Zyvox)

The first example of a new class of antibiotics called the oxazolidinones. It is a reversible, non-selective MAOI. It is highly effective against all Gram +ve organisms including MRSA, penicillin resistant pneumococci and VRE (vancomycin-resistant enterococci). Emergence of resistance during therapy has been uncommon to date. Linezolid is a useful alternative to the glycopeptides (teicoplanin and vancomycin) in patients with renal impairment as it is not known to be nephrotoxic, and does not require therapeutic dosage monitoring. The oral route (tablets or suspension) has good bioavailability and is therefore given at the same dose as the IV formulation.

Uses
- Community acquired pneumonia
- Nosocomial pneumonia (combined with antibiotic active against Gram −ve organisms)
- Severe infections due to MRSA
- Complicated skin and soft tissue infections
- Infections due to VRE

Contraindications
Concurrent use of MAOIs (Types A or B) or within two weeks of taking such drugs.

Administration
Recommended duration of treatment is 10–14 consecutive days. Safety and effectiveness of Linezolid when administered for periods longer than 28 days have not been established.

Oral: 600 mg 12 hourly
Also available as suspension (100 mg/5 ml) 30 ml 12 hourly
IV: 600 mg (300 ml bag containing 2 mg/ml solution) 12 hourly infused over 30–120 min

Monitor FBC weekly (risk of reversible myelosupression)

How not to use linezolid
Currently licensed for up to 14 days therapy only (risk of myelosuppression may increase with longer duration)

Adverse effects
Oral and vaginal candidiasis
Diarrhoea
Nausea
Reversible myelosupression
Headaches

Cautions
Severe renal failure
Unless close BP monitoring possible, avoid in uncontrolled hypertension, phaeochromocytoma, carcinoid tumour, thyrotoxicosis and patients on SSRIs, tricyclic antidepressants, pethidine, buspirone or sympathomimetics or dopaminergic drugs.

Organ failure
Renal: no dose adjustment required
Hepatic: no dose adjustment required

LIOTHYRONINE

Liothyronine has a similar action to levothyroxine but has a more rapid effect and is more rapidly metabolised. Its effects develop after a few hours and disappear within 1–2 days of discontinuing treatment. It is available both as a tablet for oral administration and as a solution for slow intravenous injection. It is useful in severe hypothyroid states when a rapid response is desired. If adverse effects occur due to excessive dosage, withhold for 1–2 days and restart at a lower dose. The injectable form is useful in patients unable to absorb enterally.

Uses
Replacement for those unable to absorb enterally
Hypothyroid states, including coma

Contraindications
Thyrotoxicosis

Administration
Hypothyroid coma: 5–20 microgram slow IV, 12 hourly. Give concurrent hydrocortisone 100 mg IV, 8 hourly, especially if pituitary hypothyroidism suspected.
Replacement for those unable to absorb enterally: 5–20 micrograms slow IV, 12 hourly, depending on the normal dose of levothyroxine.

Equivalent dose:

Oral levothyroxine	IV liothyronine
200 micrograms daily	20 micrograms 12 hourly
150 micrograms daily	15 micrograms 12 hourly
100 micrograms daily	10 micrograms 12 hourly
50 micrograms daily	5 micrograms 12 hourly

Monitor:
ECG before and during treatment
TSH (T3 and T4 may be unreliable in the critically ill)
Normal range: TSH 0.5–5.7 mU/l, T3 1.2–3.0 nmol/l, T4 70–140 nmol/l

How not to use liothyronine
Rapid IV bolus

L

Adverse effects
Tachycardia
Arrhythmias
Angina
Muscle cramps
Restlessness
Tremors

Cautions
Panhypopituitarism or predisposition to adrenal insufficiency (give hydro-cortisone before liothyronine)
IHD (may worsen ischaemia)

LOPERAMIDE

Reduces GI motility by direct effect on nerve endings and intramural ganglia within the intestinal wall. Very little is absorbed systemically.

Uses
Acute or chronic diarrhoea

Contraindications
Bowel obstruction
Toxic megacolon
Pseudomembranous colitis

Administration
Orally: 4 mg, then 2 mg after each loose stool to a maximum of 16 mg/day
Available in 2 mg capsules and 1 mg/5 ml syrup
Stools should be cultured

Adverse effects
Bloating
Abdominal pain

LORAZEPAM (Ativan)

Lorazepam may now be the preferred first-line drug for stopping status epilepticus (p. 209). Although it may have a slower onset of action, it carries a lower risk of cardiorespiratory depression (respiratory arrest, hypotension) than diazepam as it is less lipid soluble. Lorazepam also has a longer duration of anticonvulsant activity compared with diazepam (6–12 h versus 15–30 min after a single bolus).

Uses
Termination of epileptic fit

Contraindications
Airway obstruction

Administration
- IV: 4 mg over 2 min, repeated after 10 min if no response
- IM: 4 mg, dilute with 1 ml of WFI or 0.9% saline

Ampoules stored in refrigerator between 0°C and 4°C

How not to use lorazepam
IM injection – painful and unpredictable absorption, only use when IV route not possible

Adverse effects
Respiratory depression and apnoea
Drowsiness
Hypotension and bradycardia

Cautions
Airway obstruction with further neurological damage
Enhanced and prolonged sedative effect in the elderly
Additive effects with other CNS depressants

Organ failure
CNS: enhanced and prolonged sedative effect
Respiratory: ↑ respiratory depression
Hepatic: enhanced and prolonged sedative effect. Can precipitate coma
Renal: enhanced and prolonged sedative effect

100 mls NaCl
over 30 mins

MAGNESIUM SULPHATE

Like potassium, magnesium is one of the major cations of the body responsible for neurotransmission and neuromuscular excitability. Regulation of magnesium balance is mainly by the kidneys.

Hypomagnesaemia may result from failure to supply adequate intake, from excess NG drainage or suctioning, or in acute pancreatitis. It is usually accompanied by a loss of potassium. The patient may become confused, irritable with muscle twitching.

Hypomagnesaemia should also be suspected in association with other fluid and electrolyte disturbances when the patient develops unexpected neurological features or cardiac arrhythmias.

Magnesium sulphate has long been the mainstay of treatment for pre-eclampsia/eclampsia in America, but the practice in the UK until recently has been to use more specific anti-convulsant and antihypertensive agents. A large international collaborative trial shows a lower risk of recurrent convulsions in eclamptic mothers given magnesium sulphate compared with those given diazepam or phenytoin.

Normal serum magnesium concentration: 0.7–1.0 mmol/l
Therapeutic range for pre-eclampsia/eclampsia: 2.0–3.5 mmol/l

Uses
Hypomagnesaemia
Hypomagnesaemia associated with cardiac arrhythmias
Pre-eclampsia
Anticonvulsant in eclampsia
Cardiac arrest (p. 198)

Contraindications
Hypocalcaemia (further $\downarrow Ca^{2+}$)
Heart block (risk of arrhythmias)
Oliguria

Administration
Magnesium sulphate solution for injection

Concentration (%)	g/ml	mEq/ml	mmol/ml
10	0.1	0.8	0.4
25	0.25	2	1
50	0.5	4	2

1 g = 8 mEq = 4 mmol

- Hypomagnesaemia

IV infusion: 10 mmol magnesium sulphate made up to 50 ml with 5% dextrose
Do not give at >30 mmol/h
Repeat until plasma level is normal
Concentrations <20% are suitable for peripheral IV administration

- Hypomagnesaemia associated with cardiac arrhythmias

IV infusion: 20 mmol diluted in 100 ml 5% dextrose, given over 1 h
Do not give at >30 mmol/h
Repeat until plasma level is normal
Concentrations <20% are suitable for peripheral IV administration

- Pre-eclampsia/eclampsia

Loading dose: 4 g (8 ml 50% solution) diluted in 250 ml 0.9% saline IV, over 10 min
Maintenance: 1 g per h IV, as necessary. Add 10 ml 50% magnesium sulphate to 40 ml 0.9% saline and infuse at 10 ml/h
Newborn – monitor for hyporeflexia and respiratory depression

Monitor: BP, respiratory rate

ECG

Tendon reflexes

Renal function

Serum magnesium level

Maintain urine output >30 ml/h

How not to use magnesium sulphate
Rapid IV infusion can cause respiratory or cardiac arrest
IM injections (risk of abscess formation)

Adverse effects

Related to serum level:

- 4.0–6.5 mmol/l

  Nausea and vomiting

  Somnolence

  Double vision

  Slurred speech

  Loss of patellar reflex

- 6.5–7.5 mmol/l

  Muscle weakness and paralysis

  Respiratory arrest

  Bradycardia, arrhythmias and hypotension

- >10 mmol/l

  Cardiac arrest

Plasma concentrations >4.0 mmol/l cause toxicity which may be treated with calcium gluconate 1 g IV (10 ml 10%)

Cautions

Oliguria and renal impairment (↑ risk of toxic levels)

Potentiates both depolarizing and non-depolarizing muscle relaxants

Organ failure

Renal: reduce dose and slower infusion rate, closer monitoring for signs of toxicity

Renal replacement therapy

Removed by HD/HF/PD. Accumulates in renal failure; monitor levels

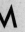

MANNITOL

An alcohol capable of causing an osmotic diuresis. Available as 10% and 20% solutions. Crystallization may occur at low temperatures. It has a rapid onset of action and duration of action is up to 4 h. Rapid infusion of mannitol increases the cardiac output and the BP.

Uses
Cerebral oedema
Preserve renal function peri-operatively in jaundiced patients
To initiate diuresis in transplanted kidneys
Rhabdomyolysis

Contraindications
Congestive cardiac failure
Pulmonary oedema (acute expansion of blood volume)
↑ Intravascular volume (further ↑ intravascular volume)

Administration
• Cerebral oedema

IV infusion: 0.5–1.0 g/kg as a 20% solution, given over 30 min

Weight (kg)	Volume of 20% mannitol at 0.5 g/kg (ml)
60	150
70	175
80	200
90	225
100	250

100 ml 20% solution = 20 g

• Jaundice

Pre-operative:
Insert urinary catheter
1000 ml 0.9% saline over 1 h, 2 h before surgery
250 ml 20% mannitol over 30 min, 1 h before surgery
Per-operative:
200–500 ml 20% mannitol if urine output <60 ml/h
0.9% saline to match urine output

• Kidney transplant

IV infusion: 0.5–1.0 g/kg over 30 min, given with frusemide 40 mg IV on reperfusion of transplanted kidney

• Rhabdomyolysis

IV infusion: 0.5–1.0 g/kg as a 20% solution over 30–60 min

How not to use mannitol
Do not give in the same line as blood
Only give mannitol to reduce ICP when the cause is likely to be relieved surgically (rebound increase in ICP)

Adverse effects
Fluid overload
Hyponatraemia and hypokalaemia
Rebound ↑ ICP

Cautions
Extravasation (thrombophlebitis)

Organ failure
Cardiac: worsens
Renal: fluid overload

Renal replacement therapy
No further dose modification is required during renal replacement therapy

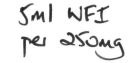

5ml WFI per 250mg

MEROPENEM (Meronem)

Meropenem is similar to imipenem but is stable to the renal enzyme dehydropeptidase−1, which inactivates imipenem. Meropenem has an extremely wide spectrum of activity, including most aerobic and anaerobic Gram −ve and +ve bacteria (but not MRSA).

Uses
- Meningitis
- Mixed aerobic/anaerobic infections
- Presumptive therapy of a wide range of severe infections prior to availability of sensitivities
- Febrile neutropenia

Contraindications
Hypersensitivity to meropenem
Infections caused by MRSA

Administration
- IV: 0.5–1.0 g 8 hourly, given over 5 min

Reconstitute with 10 ml WFI

- IV infusion: 0.5–1.0 g 8 hourly, give over 15–30 min

For meningitis, increase to 2 g 8 hourly
In renal impairment:

CC (ml/min)	Dose*	Interval (h)
20–50	1 unit dose	12
10–20	0.5 unit dose	12
<10	0.5 unit dose	24

*Based on unit doses of 0.5, 1 or 2 g

Monitor:
    FBC
    LFT

Adverse effects
Thrombophlebitis
Hypersensitivity reactions
Positive Coombs' test
Reversible thrombocythaemia, thrombocytopenia, eosinophilia and neutropenia
Abnormal LFT (↑ bilirubin, transaminases and alkaline phosphatase)

Cautions
Hypersensitivity to penicillins and cephalosporins
Hepatic impairment
Renal impairment
Concurrent use of nephrotoxic drugs

Organ failure
Hepatic: worsens
Renal: reduce dose

Renal replacement therapy
Removed by HD and probably by HF. For high clearance techniques it is probably sensible to dose as for CC 10–25 ml/min. Clearance by PD not likely to achieve clinical significance

MEROPENEM (Meronem)

METHYLPREDNISOLONE

Methylprednisolone is a potent corticosteroid with anti-inflammatory activity at least five times that of hydrocortisone. It has greater glucocorticoid activity and insignificant mineralocorticoid activity, making it particularly suitable for conditions where sodium and water retention would be a disadvantage. Corticosteroids have been suggested to reduce lung inflammation in ARDS. The fibroproliferative phase occurs between 7 and 14 days from the onset of ARDS. There are no controlled trials at present to show any benefit from this practice.

Uses
Fibroproliferative phase of ARDS (unlicensed)

Adjunct in *Pneumocystis carinni* pneumonia (see co-trimoxazole and pentamidine)

Contraindications
Systemic infection (unless specific anti-microbial therapy given)

Administration
• Fibroproliferative phase of ARDS (unlicensed)

IV infusion: 250 mg–1 g daily for up to 3 days, then dose reduced gradually

• Adjunct in *Pneumocystis carinii* pneumonia (see co-trimoxazole and pentamidine)

IV infusion: 1 g daily for 5 days, then dose reduced to complete 21 days of treatment
The steroid should be started at the same time as the co-trimoxazole or pentamidine and should be withdrawn before the antibiotic treatment is complete.
Reconstitute with WFI. Make up to 50 ml 0.9% saline or 5% dextrose, give over at least 30 min

How not to use methylprednisolone
Do not give by rapid IV injection (hypotension, arrhythmia, cardiac arrest)
Avoid live virus vaccinations

Adverse effects

Prolonged use may also lead to the following problems:

- Increased susceptibility to infections
- Impaired wound healing
- Peptic ulceration
- Muscle weakness (proximal myopathy)
- Osteoporosis
- Hyperglycaemia

Cautions

Diabetes mellitus
Concurrent use of NSAID (increased risk of GI bleeding)

METOCLOPRAMIDE

Metoclopramide acts by promoting gastric emptying, increasing gut motility, and has anti-emetic effect. It raises the threshold of the chemoreceptor trigger zone. In high-doses it has 5-HT$_3$ antagonist action.

Uses
Anti-emetic
Promotes gastric emptying
Increases lower oesophageal sphincter tone

Give neat centrally

Administration
- IV/IM: 10 mg 8 hourly

How not to use metoclopramide
Orally not appropriate if actively vomiting
Rapid IV bolus (hypotension)

Make up to 5 mls with NaCl

Adverse effects
Extrapyramidal movements
Neuroleptic malignant syndrome

Cautions
Increased risk of extrapyramidal side-effects occurs in the following:

- Hepatic and renal impairment
- Children, young adults (especially girls) and the very old
- Concurrent use of anti-psychotics
- Concurrent use of lithium

Treatment of acute oculogyric crises includes stopping metoclopramide (usually subside within 24 h) or giving procyclidine 5–10 mg IV (usually effective within 5 min)

Organ failure
Hepatic: reduce dose
Renal: reduce dose

Renal replacement therapy
No further dose modification is required during renal replacement therapy

METRONIDAZOLE

High activity against anaerobic bacteria and protozoa. It is also effective in the treatment of *Clostridium difficile* associated disease preferably given by the oral route. IV metronidazole may be used in patients with impaired gastric emptying and/or ileus.

Uses
- *Clostridium difficile* associated diarrhoea
- Anaerobic infections
- Protozoal infections (*Trichomonas vaginalis*, *Giardia intestinalis* and amoebic dysentery)
- Bacterial vaginosis
- Eradication of *Helicobacter pylori*

Administration
- *Clostridium difficile* associated diarrhoea

Orally: 400 mg 8 hourly
IV: 500 mg 8 hourly

- Anaerobic infections

IV: 500 mg 8 hourly
PR: 1 g 8 hourly

Adverse effects
Nausea and vomiting
Unpleasant taste
Rashes, urticaria and angioedema
Darkening of urine
Peripheral neuropathy (prolonged treatment)

Cautions
Hepatic impairment
Disulfiram-like reaction with alcohol

MIDAZOLAM

Midazolam is a water-soluble benzodiazepine with a short duration of action (elimination half-life 1–4 h). However, prolonged coma has been reported in some critically ill patients usually after prolonged infusions. Midazolam is metabolized to the metabolite α-hydroxy midazolam, which is rapidly conjugated. Accumulation of midazolam after prolonged sedation has been observed in critically ill patients. In renal failure, the glucuronide may also accumulate causing narcosis.

Uses
Sedation
Anxiolysis

Contraindications
As an analgesic
Airway obstruction

Administration
- IV bolus: 2.5–5 mg PRN
- IV infusion: 0.5–6 mg/h

Administer neat or diluted in 5% dextrose or 0.9% saline
Titrate dose to level of sedation required
Stop or reduce infusion each day until patient awakes, when it is restarted. Failure to assess daily will result in delayed awakening when infusion is finally stopped
Time to end effects after infusion: 30 min to 2 h (but see below)

How not to use midazolam
The use of flumazenil after prolonged use may produce confusion, toxic psychosis, convulsions, or a condition resembling delirium tremens.

Adverse effects
Residual and prolonged sedation
Respiratory depression and apnoea
Hypotension

Given neat 50 mg bottles

Cautions

Enhanced and prolonged sedative effect results from interaction with:

- opioid analgesics
- antidepressants
- antihistamines
- α-blockers
- anti-psychotics

Enhanced effect in the elderly and in patients with hypovolaemia, vaso-constriction, or hypothermia.

Midazolam is metabolized by the hepatic microsomal enzyme system (cytochrome P450s). Induction of the P450 enzyme system by another drug can gradually increase the rate of metabolism of midazolam, resulting in lower plasma concentrations and a reduced effect. Conversely inhibition of the metabolism of midazolam results in a higher plasma concentration and an increased effect. Examples of enzyme inducers and inhibitors are listed on p. 191.

There is now available a specific antagonist, flumazenil (p. 87)

Organ failure

CNS: sedative effects increased
Cardiac: exaggerated hypotension
Respiratory: ↑ respiratory depression
Hepatic: enhanced and prolonged sedative effect. Can precipitate coma
Renal: increased cerebral sensitivity

Renal replacement therapy

No further dose modification is required during renal replacement therapy

MILRINONE

Milrinone is a selective phosphodiesterase III inhibitor resulting in ↑ CO, and ↓ PCWP and SVR, without significant ↑ in HR and myocardial oxygen consumption. It produces slight enhancement in AV node conduction and may ↑ ventricular rate in uncontrolled AF/atrial flutter.

Uses
Severe congestive cardiac failure

Contraindications
Severe aortic or pulmonary stenosis (exaggerated hypotension)
Hypertrophic obstructive cardiomyopathy (exaggerated hypotension)

Administration
- IV infusion: 50 microgram/kg loading dose over 10 min, then maintain on 0.375–0.75 microgram/kg/min to a maximum haemodynamic effect

Requires direct arterial BP monitoring
Adjustment of the infusion rate should be made according to haemodynamic response
Available in 10 ml ampoules containing 10 mg milrinone (1 mg/ml)
Dilute this 10 ml solution with 40 ml 0.9% saline or 5% dextrose giving a solution containing milrinone 200 microgram/ml

Dose (microgram/kg/min)	Infusion rate (ml/kg/h)
0.375	0.11
0.4	0.12
0.5	0.15
0.6	0.18
0.7	0.21
0.75	0.22

Maximum daily dose: 1.13 mg/kg

In renal impairment:

CC (ml/min)	Dose (microgram/kg/min)
20–50	0.28–0.43
<10–20	0.23–0.28
<10	0.2–0.23

How not to use milrinone
Furosemide and bumetanide should not be given in the same line as milrinone (precipitation)

Adverse effects
Hypotension
Arrhythmias

Cautions
Uncontrolled AF/atrial flutter

Organ failure
Renal: reduce dose

Renal replacement therapy
No further dose modification is required during renal replacement therapy

MORPHINE

Morphine is the standard opioid to which others are compared and remains a valuable drug for the treatment of acute, severe pain. Peak effect after IV bolus is 15 min. Duration of action is between 2 and 3 h. Both liver and kidney function are responsible for morphine elimination. The liver mainly metabolizes it. One of the principal metabolites, M6G, is also a potent opioid agonist and may accumulate in renal failure.

Uses
Relief of severe pain
To facilitate mechanical ventilation
Acute left ventricular failure – by relieving anxiety and producing vasodilatation

Contraindications
Airway obstruction
Pain caused by biliary colic

Administration
- IV bolus: 2.5 mg every 15 min PRN
- IV infusion rate: 1–5 mg/h

Dilute in 5% glucose or 0.9% saline
Stop or reduce infusion each day and restart when first signs of discomfort appear. Failure to assess daily will result in overdosage and difficulty in weaning patient from ventilation

- If the patient is conscious the best method is to give an infusion pump they can control (PCAS): 60 mg made up to 60 ml with 0.9% saline; IV bolus: 1 mg; lockout: 3–10 min

How not to use morphine
In combination with an opioid partial agonist, e.g. buprenorphine (antagonizes opioid effects)

Adverse effects
Respiratory depression and apnoea
Hypotension and tachycardia
Nausea and vomiting
Delayed gastric emptying
Reduce intestinal mobility
Biliary spasm
Constipation
Urinary retention
Histamine release
Tolerance
Pulmonary oedema

Cautions
Enhanced and prolonged effect when used in patients with renal failure, the elderly, and in patients with hypovolaemia and hypothermia
Enhanced sedative and respiratory depression from interaction with:

- benzodiazepines
- antidepressants
- anti-psychotics

Head injury and neurosurgical patients (may exacerbate $\uparrow$ ICP as a result of $\uparrow$ $PaCO_2$)

Organ failure
CNS: sedative effects increased
Respiratory: $\uparrow$ respiratory depression
Hepatic: can precipitate coma
Renal: increased cerebral sensitivity. M6G accumulates

Renal replacement therapy
Removed by HD/HF but significant only with high clearance techniques – also removes active metabolite M6G which accumulates in renal failure. Titrate to response. Not significantly removed by PD.

NALOXONE

This is a specific opioid antagonist. The elimination half-life is 60–90 min, with a duration of action between 30 and 45 min.

Uses
Reversal of opioid adverse effects – respiratory depression, sedation, pruritus and urinary retention
As a diagnostic test of opioid overdose in an unconscious patient

Contraindications
Patients physically dependent on opioids

Administration
- Reversal of opioid overdose: 200 microgram IV bolus, repeat every 2–3 min until desired response, up to a total of 2 mg
- Reversal of spinal opioid induced pruritus: dilute 200 microgram in 10 ml WFI. Give 20 microgram boluses every 5 min until symptoms resolve

Titrate dose carefully in postoperative patients to avoid sudden return of severe pain

How not to use naloxone
Large doses given quickly

Adverse effects
- Arrhythmias
- Hypertension

Cautions
Withdrawal reactions in patients on long-term opioid for medical reasons or in addicts
Postoperative patients – return of pain and severe haemodynamic disturbances (hypertension, VT/VF, pulmonary oedema)

Organ failure
Hepatic: delayed elimination

NEOSTIGMINE

Neostigmine is a cholinesterase inhibitor leading to prolongation of ACh action. This will enhance parasympathetic activity in the gut and increase intestinal motility. When used for acute colonic pseudo-obstruction, organic obstruction of the gut must first be excluded and it should not be used shortly after bowel anastomosis (Ponec RJ, et al. *New England Journal of Medicine* 1999; 341: 137–41). Colonic pseudo-obstruction, which is the massive dilation of the colon in the absence of mechanical obstruction, can develop after surgery or severe illness. Most cases respond to conservative treatment. In patients who do not respond, colonic decompression is often performed to prevent ischaemia and perforation of the bowel. Colonoscopy in these patients is not always successful and can be accompanied by complications such as perforation.

Uses
Colonic pseudo-obstruction (unlicensed)

Administration
- IV bolus: 2.5 mg, repeated 3 h later if no response to initial dose

Monitor ECG (may need to give atropine or other anticholinergic drugs to counteract symptomatic bradycardia)

Contraindications
Mechanical bowel obstruction
Urinary obstruction

How not to use neostigmine
It should not be used shortly after bowel anastomosis

Adverse effects
Increased sweating
Excess salivation
Nausea and vomiting
Abdominal cramp
Diarrhoea
Bradycardia
Hypotension
These muscarinic side-effects are antagonized by atropine

Cautions
Asthma

Organ failure
Renal: reduce dose

Renal replacement therapy
No further dose modification is required during renal replacement therapy

NIMODIPINE

A calcium-channel blocker with smooth muscle relaxant effect preferentially in the cerebral arteries. Its use is confined to prevention of vascular spasm after subarachnoid haemorrhage. Nimodipine is used in conjunction with the 'triple H' regime of hypertension, hypervolaemia and haemodilution to a haematocrit of 30–33.

Uses
Subarachnoid haemorrhage

Administration
• IV infusion

1 mg/h, ↑ to 2 mg/h if BP not severely ↓
If <70 kg or BP unstable start at 0.5 mg/h
Ready prepared solution – do not dilute
But administer into a running infusion (40 ml/h) of 0.9% saline or 5% dextrose, via a central line
Continue for between 5 and 14 days
Use only polyethylene or polypropylene infusion sets
Protect from light

10 mg in 50 ml vial (0.02%)
0.5 mg/hr = 2.5 ml/hr
1 mg/hr = 5 ml/hr
2 mg/hr = 10 ml/hr

• Orally (prophylaxis)

60 mg every 4 h for 21 days

How not to use nimodipine
Avoid PVC infusion sets
Do not use peripheral venous access
Do not give nimodipine tablets and IV infusion concurrently
Avoid concurrent use of other calcium-channel blockers, b-blockers or nephrotoxic drugs

Adverse effects
Hypotension (vasodilatation)
Transient ↑ liver enzymes with IV use

Cautions
Hypotension (may be counter-productive by ↓ cerebral perfusion)
Cerebral oedema or severely ↑ ICP
Renal impairment

make up with 5% dextrose
T.V 50mls

40 mls Dextro
4 ml Nora
Single
Strength

NORADRENALINE

α_1 effect predominates over its β_1 effect, raising the BP by increasing the SVR. It increases the myocardial oxygen requirement without increasing coronary blood flow. Noradrenaline (norepinephrine) reduces renal, hepatic, and muscle blood flow. But in septic shock, noradrenaline may increase renal blood flow and enhance urine production by increasing perfusion pressure. Acute renal failure secondary to inadequate renal perfusion is a common form of kidney failure seen in the ICU. Once intravascular volume has been restored, the MAP should be restored to a level that optimally preserves renal perfusion pressure i.e. above 75–80 mmHg (or higher in previously hypertensive patients).

Uses
Septic shock, with low SVR

Contraindications
Hypovolaemic shock
Acute myocardial ischaemia or MI

Administration
• Usual dose range: 0.01–0.4 microgram/kg/min IV infusion via a central vein

Initially start at a higher rate than intended to increase the BP more rapidly and then reduce rate
4 mg made up to 50 ml 5% dextrose (80 microgram/ml)

Dosage chart (ml/h)

Weight (kg)	Dose (microgram/kg/min)				
	0.02	0.05	0.1	0.15	0.2
50	0.8	1.9	3.8	5.6	7.5
60	0.9	2.3	4.5	6.8	9
70	1.1	2.6	5.3	7.9	10.5
80	1.2	3	6	9	12
90	1.4	3.4	6.8	10.1	13.5
100	1.5	3.8	7.5	11.3	15
110	1.7	4.1	8.3	12.4	16.5
120	1.8	4.5	9	13.5	18

NORADRENALINE

INOTROPE

139

How not to use noradrenaline

In the absence of haemodynamic monitoring
Do not use a peripheral vein (risk of extravasation)
Do not connect to CVP lumen used for monitoring pressure (surge of drug during flushing of line)

Adverse effects

Bradycardia
Hypertension
Arrhythmias
Myocardial ischaemia

Cautions

Hypertension
Heart disease
If extravasation of noradrenaline occurs – phentolamine 10 mg in 15 ml 0.9% saline should be infiltrated into the ischaemic area with a 23-G needle

NYSTATIN

Nystatin is a polyene antifungal which is not absorbed when given orally and is too toxic for IV use.

Uses
Oral candida infection
Suppression of gut carriage of candida
Topical therapy of genital candida infections

Administration
• Oral candidiasis

1 ml (100,000 units) 6 hourly, holding in mouth

• Prophylaxis

Orally: 1 million units daily

How not to use nystatin
IV too toxic

Adverse effects
Rash
Oral irritation

OCTREOTIDE

Octreotide is an analogue of somatostatin. It is used to provide relief from symptoms associated with carcinoid tumours and acromegaly. It may also be used for the prevention of complications following pancreatic surgery. For patients undergoing pancreatic surgery, the peri and post-operative administration of octreotide reduces the incidence of typical post-operative complications (e.g. pancreatic fistula, abscess and subsequent sepsis, post-operative acute pancreatitis). Octreotide exerts an inhibiting effect on gallbladder motility, bile acid secretion and bile flow and there is an acknowledged association with the development of gallstones in prolonged usage.

Uses
Prevention of complications following pancreatic surgery
Pancreatic leak (unlicensed)

Administration
• Prevention of complications following pancreatic surgery

SC or IV: 100 microgram 8 hourly for 7 days, starting on the day of operation at least one hour before laparotomy

• Pancreatic leak

SC or IV: 100 microgram 8 hourly

To reduce pain and irritation on injection, allow solution to reach room temperature and rotate injection site
IV dose should be diluted with 5 ml 0.9% saline

Stored in fridge between 2–8°C

How not to use octreotide
Abrupt withdrawal (biliary colic and pancreatitis)
Dilution with solution containing glucose is not recommended

Adverse effects
GI disturbances (nausea, vomiting, pain, bloating, diarrhoea)
Pain and irritation at injection site (allow solution to reach room temperature and rotate injection sites)
Elevated LFTs
Gall stone formation with prolonged use

Cautions
Growth hormone-secreting pituitary tumour (may increase in size)
Insulinoma (hypoglycaemia)
Requirement for insulin and oral hypoglycaemic drugs may be reduced in diabetes mellitus

Organ failure
Hepatic: reduce dose

OMEPRAZOLE

Omeprazole is a proton pump inhibitor, which inhibits gastric acid production by the gastric parietal cells. Following endoscopic treatment of
bleeding peptic ulcers, omeprazole given intravenous for 72 hours has
been shown to reduce the risk of rebleeding (*NEJM* 2000; **343:** 310–6).

Uses
Bleeding peptic ulcers, after endoscopic treatment of bleeding
(unlicensed)

Administration
• Bleeding peptic ulcers, after endoscopic treatment of bleeding

IV: Initial 80 mg IV loading dose given over 1 hour, followed by 8 mg/h
IV infusion for 72 hours
Reconstitute with either 0.9% saline or 5% dextrose

See appendix G

Adverse effects
GI disturbances (nausea, vomiting, abdominal pain, diarrhoea and
constipation)
Paraesthesia
Agitation
Liver dysfunction
Hyponatraemia

100mls

Cautions
Severe hepatic disease (risk of encephalopathy)
Pregnancy (toxic in animal studies)
May mask symptoms of gastric cancer

Dextrose

Organ failure
Hepatic: reduce dose

Protects the stomach.

Give over 30 mins

ONDANSETRON

A specific 5-HT_3 antagonist.

Uses
Severe postoperative nausea and vomiting
Highly emetogenic chemotherapy

Administration
- Initial dose: 4 mg slow IV over 15 min
- Followed by continuous IV infusion of 1 mg/h for up to 24 h

Dilution: 24 mg ondansetron made up to 48 ml with 0.9% saline or 5% dextrose
Rate of infusion: 2 ml/h

How not to use ondansetron
Do not give rapidly as IV bolus

Adverse effects
Headaches
Flushing
Constipation
Increases in liver enzymes (transient)

Cautions
Hepatic impairment

Organ failure
Hepatic: reduced clearance (moderate or severe liver disease: not >8 mg daily)

PANCURONIUM

A non-depolarizing neuromuscular blocker with a long duration of action (1–2 h). It is largely excreted unchanged by the kidneys. It causes a 20% increase in HR and BP. It may be a suitable choice in the hypotensive patient, although the tachycardia induced may not be desirable if the HR is already high, e.g. hypovolaemia, septic shock.

Uses

Patients where prolonged muscle relaxation is desirable, e.g. intractable status asthmaticus

Contraindications

Airway obstruction
To facilitate tracheal intubation in patients at risk of regurgitation
Renal and hepatic failure (prolonged paralysis)
Severe muscle atrophy
Tetanus (sympathomimetic effects)

Administration

* Initial dose: 50–100 mcg/kg IV bolus

* Incremental doses: 20 mcg/kg, every 1–2 h

Monitor with peripheral nerve stimulator

How not to use pancuronium

As part of a rapid sequence induction
In the conscious patient
By persons not trained to intubate trachea

Adverse effects

Tachycardia and hypertension

Cautions

Breathing circuit (disconnection)
Prolonged use (disuse muscle atrophy)

Organ failure

Hepatic: prolonged paralysis
Renal: prolonged paralysis

Renal replacement therapy

No further dose modification is required during renal replacement therapy

P

PARACETAMOL

The efficacy of single-dose IV paracetamol as a postoperative analgesic has been confirmed by many studies. The IV formulation provides a more predicable plasma concentration and has a potency slightly less than a standard dose of morphine or the NSAIDs. The mechanism of action remains unclear as, unlike opioids and NSAIDs respectively; paracetamol has no known endogenous binding sites and does not inhibit peripheral cyclooxygenase activity significantly. There is increasing evidence of a central antinociceptive effect, and potential mechanisms for this include inhibition of a central nervous system COX-2, inhibition of a putative central cyclooxygenase 'COX-3' that is selectively susceptible to paracetamol, and modulation of inhibitory descending serotinergic pathways. Paracetamol has also been shown to prevent prostaglandin production at the cellular transcriptional level, independent of cyclooxygenase activity.

The availability of intravenous paracetamol (*Perfalgan*) will enhance and extend the use of this drug as a fundamental component of multimodal analgesia after surgery and in critical ill patients who are not able to absorb enterally.

Uses
Mild to moderate pain
Fever

Administration
Oral or PR: 0.5–1 g every 4–6 hours; maximum of 4 g daily
IV infusion: 1 g (100 ml) given over 15 min, every 4–6 hours; maximum of 4 g daily

How not to use paracetamol
Do not exceed 4 g/day

Adverse effects
Hypotension with IV infusion
Liver damage with overdose

Cautions
Hepatic impairment
Renal impairment
Alcohol dependence

Organ failure
Hepatic: avoid large doses (dose-related toxicity)
Renal: increase IV infusion dose interval to every 6 hours if creatinine clearance <30 ml/min

PENTAMIDINE

Pentamidine isetionate given by intravenous route is an alternative for patients with severe *Pneumocystis carinii* (now renamed *Pneumocystis jirovecii*) pneumonia unable to tolerate co-trimoxazole, or who have not responded to it. Pentamidine isetionate is a toxic drug and personnel handling the drug must be adequately protected. Nebulised pentamidine may be used for mild disease and for prophylaxis. Thin walled air-containing cysts (pneumatoceles) and pneumathoraces are more common in patients receiving nebulised pentamidine as prophylaxis. Adverse effects, sometimes severe, are more common with pentamidine than co-trimoxazole.

Uses
Alternative treatment for severe *Pneumocystis carinii* pneumonia (PCP).

Administration
• IV infusion: 4 mg/kg every 24 h for at least 14 days

Dilute in 250 ml 5% dextrose, given over 1–2 h

In renal impairment:

CC (ml/min)	Dose (mg/kg)	Interval (h)
10–50	4	36
<10	4	48

Adjuvant corticosteroid has been shown to improve survival. The steroid should be started at the same time as the pentamidine and should be withdrawn before the antibiotic treatment is complete. Oral prednisolone 50–80 mg daily or IV hydrocortisone 100 mg 6 hourly or IV dexamethasone 8 mg 6 hourly or IV methylprednisolone 1 g for 5 days, then dose reduced to complete 21 days of treatment.

How not to use pentamidine
Nebulized route not recommended in severe PCP ($\downarrow$ PaO_2)
Concurrent use of both co-trimoxazole and pentamidine is not of benefit and may increase the incidence of serious side-effects

Adverse effects
Acute renal failure (usually isolated $\uparrow$ serum creatinine)
Leucopenia, thrombocytopenia
Severe hypotension
Hypoglycaemia
Pancreatitis
Arrhythmias

Cautions
Blood disorders
Hypotension
Renal/hepatic impairment

Organ failure
Renal: reduce dose

Renal replacement therapy
No further dose modification is required during renal replacement therapy

PETHIDINE

Pethidine has one-tenth the analgesic potency of morphine. The duration of action is between 2 and 4 h. It has atropine-like actions and relaxes smooth muscles. The principal metabolite is norpethidine, which can cause fits. In renal failure and after infusions this metabolite can accumulate and cause seizures.

Uses

It may be indicated in controlling pain from pancreatitis, secondary to gallstones, and after surgical procedure involving bowel anastomosis where it is claimed to cause less increase in the intraluminal pressures. It produces less release of histamine than morphine, and may be preferable in asthmatics.

Contraindications
Airway obstruction
Concomitant use of MAOI

Administration
• IV bolus: 10–50 mg PRN

Duration of action: 2–3 h

• PCAS: 600 mg in 60 ml 0.9% saline

IV bolus: 10 mg, lockout 5–10 min

How not to use pethidine
In combination with an opioid partial agonist, e.g. buprenorphine (antagonizes opioid effects)

Adverse effects
Respiratory depression and apnoea
Hypotension and tachycardia
Nausea and vomiting
Delayed gastric emptying
Reduce intestinal mobility
Constipation
Urinary retention
Histamine release
Tolerance
Pulmonary oedema

Cautions
Enhanced sedative and respiratory depression from interaction with:

- benzodiazepines
- antidepressants
- anti-psychotics

Avoid concomitant use of and for 2 weeks after MAOI discontinued (risk of CNS excitation or depression – hypertension, hyperpyrexia, convulsions and coma)

Head injury and neurosurgical patients (may exacerbate ↑ ICP as a result of ↑ $PaCO_2$)

Organ failure
CNS: sedative effects increased
Respiratory: ↑ respiratory depression
Hepatic: enhanced and prolonged sedative effect. Can precipitate coma
Renal: increased cerebral sensitivity. Norpethidine accumulates

Renal replacement therapy
No further dose modification is required during renal replacement therapy

PHENOBARBITONE

Uses
Status epilepticus (p. 209)

Contraindications
Porphyria

Administration
• IV: 10 mg/kg (maximum daily dose 1 g)

Dilute to 10 times its own volume with WFI immediately before use. Give at <100 mg/min
Reduce dose and inject more slowly in the elderly, patients with severe hepatic and renal impairment, and in hypovolaemic and shocked patients
In obese patients, dosage should be based on lean body mass

Adverse effects
Respiratory depression
Hypotension
Bradycardia
CNS depression

Organ failure
CNS: sedative effects increased
Respiratory: ↑ respiratory depression
Hepatic: can precipitate coma
Renal: reduce dose

Renal replacement therapy
No further dose modification is required during renal replacement therapy

PHENTOLAMINE

Phentolamine is a short-acting α-blocker that produces peripheral vasodilatation by blocking both α_1- and α_2-adrenergic receptors. Pulmonary vascular resistance and pulmonary arterial pressure are decreased.

Uses
Severe hypertension associated with phaeochromocytoma

Contraindications
Hypotension

Administration
Available in 10 mg ampoules

- IV bolus: 2–5 mg, repeat PRN
- IV infusion: 0.1–2 mg/min

Dilute in 0.9% saline or 5% dextrose
Monitor pulse and BP continuously

How not to use phentolamine
Do not use adrenaline, ephedrine, isoprenaline or dobutamine to treat phentolamine-induced hypotension (β_2 effect of these sympathomimetics will predominate causing a further paradoxical $\downarrow$ BP)
Treat phentolamine-induced hypotension with noradrenaline

Adverse effects
Hypotension
Tachycardia and arrhythmias
Dizziness
Nasal congestion

Cautions
Asthma (sulphites in ampoule may lead to hypersensitivity)
IHD

PHENYTOIN

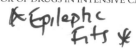 *Epileptic Fits*

P

Uses
Status epilepticus (p. 208)
Anticonvulsant prophylaxis in post-neurosurgical operations
Anti-arrhythmic – particularly for arrhythmias associated with digoxin toxicity

Contraindications
Do not use IV phenytoin in sino-atrial block, or second- and third-degree AV block

Administration
- Status epilepticus: 15 mg/kg, give at a rate not >50 mg/min (20–30 min), followed by 100 mg every 6–8 hourly for maintenance
- Anticonvulsant prophylaxis: 200–600 mg/day PO/IV
- Anti-arrhythmic: 100 mg IV every 15 min until arrhythmia stops. Maximum 15 mg/kg/day

Monitor:

ECG and BP

Serum phenytoin level (p. 193)

How not to use phenytoin
Rapid IV bolus not recommended (hypotension, arrhythmias, CNS depression)
Do not dissolve in solutions containing glucose (precipitation)
IM injection not recommended (absorption slow and erratic)
Do not give into an artery (gangrene)

Adverse effects
Nystagmus, ataxia and slurred speech
Drowsiness and confusion
Hypotension (rapid IV)
Prolonged QT interval and arrhythmias (rapid IV)
Gingival hyperplasia (long-term)
Rashes
Aplastic anaemia
Agranulocytosis
Megaloblastic anaemia
Thrombocytopenia

Cautions
Severe liver disease (reduce dose)
Metabolism subject to other enzyme inducers and inhibitors (p. 191)
Additive CNS depression with other CNS depressants

Organ failure
CNS: enhanced sedation
Hepatic: increase serum level

PHOSPHATES

Hypophosphataemia may lead to muscle weakness and is a cause of difficulty in weaning a patient from mechanical ventilation. Causes of hypophosphataemia in ICU include failure of supplementation, e.g. during TPN, use of insulin and high concentration glucose, use of loop diuretics and low dose dopamine.

Normal range: 0.8–1.4 mmol/l

Uses
Hypophosphataemia

Contraindications
Hypocalcaemia (further ↓ Ca^{2+})
Severe renal failure (risk of hyperphosphataemia)

Administration
• IV infusion: 10 mmol phosphate (K/Na) made up to 50 ml with 5% dextrose or 0.9% saline, given over 12 h

Do not give at >10 mmol over 12 h
Repeat until plasma level is normal

Available in ampoules of:

• Potassium hydrogen phosphate 5 ml 17.42% (potassium 2 mmol/ml, phosphate 1 mmol/ml)

• Sodium hydrogen phosphate 10 ml 17.91% (sodium 1 mmol/ml, phosphate 0.5 mmol/ml)

Monitor serum calcium, phosphate, potassium, and sodium daily

How not to use phosphate
Do not give rapidly

Adverse effects
Hypocalcaemia, hypomagnesaemia, hyperkalaemia, hypernatraemia
Arrhythmias
Hypotension
Ectopic calcification

Cautions
Renal impairment
Concurrent use of potassium-sparing diuretics or ACE-I with potassium phosphate may result in hyperkalaemia
Concurrent use of corticosteroids with sodium phosphate may result in hypernatraemia

Organ failure
Renal: risk of hyperphosphataemia

Renal replacement therapy
Phosphate accumulates in renal failure. Removed by HD/HF but significant only with high clearance techniques. Treat hypophosphataemia only on the basis of measured serum levels

Mix with 20 mls WFI

PIPERACILLIN + TAZOBACTAM (Tazocin)

Tazocin is a combination of piperacillin (a broad-spectrum penicillin) and tazobactam (a beta-lactamase inhibitor). It has activity against many Gram +ve, Gram −ve and anaerobic bacteria. Tazocin may act synergistically with aminoglycosides against Gram −ve organisms including *Pseudomonas aeruginosa*. However it remains susceptible to chromosomal beta lactamases expressed by Enterobacteriaceae such as *Enterobacter* spp. and *Citrobacter* spp. and is unreliable for organisms expressing extended spectrum beta-lactamases (ESBLs). Tazocin appears to have a lower propensity to cause superinfection with *Clostridium difficile* compared with fluoroquinolones and cephalosporins.

Uses
- Intra-abdominal infection
- Respiratory tract infection particularly nosocomial pneumonia
- Severe upper urinary tract infection
- Empirical therapy of a range of severe infections prior to availability of sensitivities
- Febrile neutropenia (usually combined with an aminoglycoside)

Contraindications
Penicillin hypersensitivity
Cephalosporin hypersensitivity

Administration
Reconstitute 2.25 g with 10 ml WFI
Reconstitute 4.5 g with 20 ml WFI

- IV bolus: 2.25–4.5 g 6–8 hourly, given over 3–5 min
- IV infusion: Dilute the reconstituted solution to at least 50 ml with 5% dextrose or 0.9% saline, given over 20–30 min

Infection	Dose (g)	Interval (h)
mild–moderate	2.25	8
moderate–serious	4.5	8
life-threatening	4.5	6

In renal impairment:

CC (ml/min)	Dose (g)	Interval (h)
20–80	4.5	8
<20	4.5	12

How not to use tazocin

Not for intrathecal use (encephalopathy)

Do not mix in the same syringe with an aminoglycoside (efficacy of aminoglycoside reduced)

Adverse effects

Diarrhoea

Muscle pain or weakness

Hallucination

Convulsion (high dose or renal failure)

Cautions

Owing to the sodium content (~2 mmol/g), high doses may lead to hypernatraemia

Organ failure

Renal: reduce dose

Renal replacement therapy

No further dose modification is required during renal replacement therapy

P

PIPERACILLIN + TAZOBACTAM (Tazocin)

POTASSIUM CHLORIDE

Uses
Hypokalaemia

Contraindications
Severe renal failure
Severe tissue trauma
Untreated Addison's disease

Administration
Potassium chloride 1.5 g (20 mmol K^+) in 10 ml ampoules

IV infusion: Undiluted via central line

Do not give at >20 mmol/h
Monitor serum potassium regularly
Check serum magnesium in refractory hypokalaemia

How not to use potassium
Do not infuse neat potassium chloride into a peripheral vein
Avoid extravasation and do not give IM or SC (severe pain and tissue necrosis)

Adverse effects
Muscle weakness
Arrhythmias
ECG changes

Cautions
Renal impairment
Concurrent use of potassium-sparing diuretics or ACE-I
Hypokalaemia is frequently associated with hypomagnesaemia

Organ failure
Renal: risk of hyperkalaemia

Renal replacement therapy
Potassium accumulates in renal failure. Removed by HD/HF/PD. Treat
hypokalaemia only on the basis of measured serum levels

Compatable
with Actrapid

PROCHLORPERAZINE

P

A phenothiazine that inhibits the medullary chemoreceptor trigger zone.

Uses
Nausea and vomiting

Contraindications
Parkinson's disease

Administration
• IM/IV: 12.5 mg 6 hourly
The IV route is not licensed

Adverse effects
Drowsiness
Postural hypotension, tachycardia
Extrapyramidal movements particularly in children, elderly and debilitated

Cautions
Concurrent use of other CNS depressants (enhanced sedation)

Organ failure
CNS: sedative effects increased
Hepatic: can precipitate coma
Renal: increase cerebral sensitivity

Renal replacement therapy
No further dose modification is required during renal replacement therapy

Given IV

PROPOFOL

Propofol is an IV anaesthetic induction agent that has rapidly become popular as a sedative drug in the critically ill. Its major advantages are that it has a rapid onset of action and a rapid recovery even after prolonged infusion. Propofol 1% (10 mg/ml) and 2% (20 mg/ml) are formulated in intralipid. If the patient is receiving other IV lipid concurrently, a reduction in quantity should be made to account for the amount of lipid infused as propofol. One ml propofol 1% contains 0.1 g fat and 1 kcal.

A recent study (Cremer OL, et al. *The Lancet* 2001; 357: 117–8) has suggested an association between long term (>2 days) high dose (>5 mg/kg/hour) propofol infusion used for sedation and cardiac failure in adult patients with head injuries. All the seven patients who died developed metabolic acidosis, hyperkalaemia or rhabdomyolysis. Reports of similar suspected reactions, including hyperlipidaemia and hepatomegaly were previously reported in children given propofol infusion for sedation in intensive care units, some with fatal outcome (MCA/CSM Current Problems in Pharmacovigilance 1992; 34).

Uses
Sedation, especially for weaning from other sedative agents (p. 204)
Status epilepticus (p. 208)

Contraindications
As an analgesic
Hypersensitivity to propofol, soybean oil, or egg phosphatide (egg yolk)
Sedation of ventilated children aged 16 years or younger receiving intensive care.

Administration
- IV bolus: 10–20 mg PRN
- IV infusion: up to 4 mg/kg/h

Titrate to desired level of sedation – assess daily
Measure serum triglycerides regularly
Contains no preservatives – discard after 12 h

How not to use propofol
Do not give in the same line as blood or blood products
Do not exceed recommended dose range for sedation (up to 4 mg/kg/hour)

PROPOFOL

1% & 2%.

Adverse effects
Hypotension
Bradycardia
Apnoea
Pain on injection (minimized by mixing with lignocaine 1 mg for every 10 mg propofol)
Fat overload
Convulsions and myoclonic movements

Cautions
Epilepsy
Lipid disorders (risk of fat overload)
Egg allergy (most patients are allergic to the egg albumin – not egg yolk)

Organ failure
CNS: sedative effects increased
Cardiac: exaggerated hypotension

Sedation drugs can be given on the same line

P

PROTAMINE

Available as a 1% (10 mg/ml) solution of protamine sulphate. Although it is used to neutralize the anticoagulant action of heparin, if used in excess it has an anticoagulant effect.

Uses
Neutralize the anticoagulant action of heparin

Contraindications
Hypersensitivity

Administration
One ml 1% (10 mg) protamine is required to neutralize 1000 units of heparin given in the previous 15 min
As more time elapses after the heparin injection, proportionally less protamine is required
Slow IV injection 5 ml 1% over 10 min
Ideally, the dosage should be guided by serial measurements of APTT/ ACT and the rate guided by watching the direct arterial BP

How not to use protamine
Rapid IV bolus

Adverse effects
Hypersensitivity
Rapid IV administration – pulmonary vasoconstriction, ↓ left atrial pressure and hypotension

Cautions
Hypersensitivity (severe hypotension, may respond to fluid loading)

PYRIDOSTIGMINE (Mestinon)

Pyridostigmine is a cholinesterase inhibitor leading to prolongation of ACh action. This enhances neuromuscular transmission in voluntary and involuntary muscle in myasthenia gravis.

Uses
Myasthenia gravis

Administration
• Orally: 60–240 mg 4–6 hourly (maximum daily dose: 1.2 g)

When relatively large doses are taken it may be necessary to give atropine or other anticholinergic drugs to counteract the muscarinic effects

Contraindications
Bowel obstruction
Urinary obstruction

How not to use pyridostigmine
Excessive dosage may impair neuromuscular transmission and precipitates 'cholinergic crises' by causing a depolarizing block. It is inadvisable to exceed a daily dose of 720 mg

Adverse effects
Increased sweating
Excess salivation
Nausea and vomiting
Abdominal cramp
Diarrhoea
Bradycardia
Hypotension
These muscarinic side-effects are antagonized by atropine

Cautions
Asthma

Organ failure
Renal: reduce dose

Renal replacement therapy
No further dose modification is required during renal replacement therapy

RANITIDINE

It is a specific histamine H_2-antagonist that inhibits basal and stimulated secretion of gastric acid, reducing both the volume and the pH of the secretion.

Uses
Peptic ulcer disease
Prophylaxis of stress ulceration
Premedication in patients at risk of acid aspiration

Administration
• IV bolus: 50 mg 8 hourly

Dilute to 20 ml with 0.9% saline or 5% dextrose and give over 5 min
In severe renal impairment (CC < 10 ml/min): 25 mg 8 hourly

How not to use ranitidine
Do not give rapidly as IV bolus (bradycardia, arrhythmias)

Adverse effects
Hypersensitivity reactions
Bradycardia
Transient and reversible worsening of liver function tests
Reversible leucopaenia and thrombocytopenia

Organ failure
Renal: reduce dose
Hepatic: reduce dose (increase risk of confusion)

Renal replacement therapy
No further dose modification is required during renal replacement therapy

RIFAMPICIN

Rifampicin is active against a wide range of Gram +ve and Gram −ve organisms but resistance readily emerges during therapy due to pre-existing mutants present in most bacterial populations. It must therefore be used with a second antibiotic active against the target pathogen. Its major use is for therapy of tuberculosis.

Uses
- In combination with vancomycin for:
  Penicillin resistant pneumococcal infections including meningitis
  Serious Gram +ve infections including those caused by MRSA
  Prosthetic device associated infections
- Legionnaires' disease (in combination with a macrolide antibiotic)
- Prophylaxis of meningococcal meningitis and *Haemophilus influenzae* (type b) infection
- Combination therapy for infections due to *Mycobacterium tuberculosis*

Contraindications
Porphyria
Jaundice

Administration
- Serious Gram +ve infections (in combination with vancomycin)
- Legionnaires' disease (in combination with a macrolide antibiotic)

Oral or IV: 600 mg 12 hourly

- Prophylaxis of meningococcal meningitis infection

Oral or IV: 600 mg 12 hourly for 2 days
Child 10 mg/kg (under 1 year, 5 mg/kg) 12 hourly for 2 days

- Prophylaxis of *Haemophilus influenzae* (type b) infection

Oral or IV: 600 mg once daily for 4 days
Child 1–3 months 10 mg/kg once daily for 4 days, over 3 months 20 mg/kg once daily for 4 days (maximum 600 mg daily)

IV formulations are available as *Rifadin* and *Rimactane*.
Reconstitute with the solvent provided, then dilute with 500 ml (for *Rifadin*) or 250 ml (for *Rimactane*) of 5% dextrose, 0.9% saline or Hartmann's solution, given over 2–3 hours.

Monitor: FBC, U&E, LFT

RIFAMPICIN

Adverse effects
GI symptoms (nausea, vomiting, diarrhoea)
Body secretions (urine, saliva) coloured orange-red
Abnormal LFT
Haemolytic anaemia
Thrombocytopenic purpura
Renal failure

Cautions
Discolours soft contact lenses
Women on oral contraceptive pills will need other means of contraception

Organ failure
Hepatic: avoid or do not exceed 8 mg/kg daily (impaired elimination)

SALBUTAMOL

Uses
Reverses bronchospasm

Administration
- Nebulizer: 2.5–5 mg 6 hourly, undiluted (if prolonged delivery time desirable then dilute with 0.9% saline only)

For patients with chronic bronchitis and hypercapnia, oxygen in high concentration can be dangerous, and nebulizers should be driven by air

- IV: 5 mg made up to 50 ml with 5% dextrose (100 mcg/ml)

Rate: 200–1200 mcg/h (2–12 ml/h)

How not to use salbutamol
For nebulizer: do not dilute in anything other than 0.9% saline (hypotonic solution may cause bronchospasm)

Adverse effects
Tremor
Tachycardia
Paradoxical bronchospasm (stop giving if suspected)
Potentially serious hypokalaemia (potentiated by concomitant treatment with aminophylline, steroids, diuretics and hypoxia)

Cautions
Thyrotoxicosis
In patients already receiving large doses of other sympathomimetic drugs

SPIRONOLACTONE

Spironolactone is a potassium-sparing diuretic, which acts by antagonising aldosterone. Low doses of spironolactone have been shown to benefit patients with severe congestive heart failure, who are already receiving an ACE inhibitor and a diuretic. It is also of value in the treatment of oedema and ascites in cirrhosis of the liver.

Uses
Congestive heart failure
Oedema and ascites in liver cirrhosis

Contraindications
Hyperkalaemia
Hyponatraemia
Severe renal failure
Addison's disease

Administration
- Congestive heart failure

Orally: 25–50 mg once daily

- Oedema and ascites in liver cirrhosis

Orally: 100–200 mg once daily

Monitor: serum sodium, potassium and creatinine

Adverse effects
Confusion
Hyperkalaemia
Hyponatraemia
Abnormal LFT
Gynaecomastia (usually reversible)
Rashes

Cautions
Porphyria
Renal impairment (risk of hyperkalaemia)
Concurrent use of:

    ACE inhibitor (risk of hyperkalaemia)

    Angiotensin-II antagonist (risk of hyperkalaemia)

    Digoxin (↑ plasma concentration of digoxin)

    Ciclosporin (risk of hyperkalaemia)

    Lithium (↑ plasma concentration of lithium)

Organ failure
Renal: risk of hyperkalaemia, avoid in severe renal failure
Hepatic: may precipitate encephalopathy

SUCRALFATE

A complex of aluminium hydroxide and sulphated sucrose. It acts by protecting the mucosa from acid–pepsin attack.

Uses
Prophylaxis of stress ulceration

Contraindications
Severe renal impairment (CC <10 ml/min)

Administration
• Orally: 1 g suspension 4 hourly

Stop sucralfate when enteral feed commences

How not to use sucralfate
Do not give with enteral feed (risk of bezoar formation)
Do not give ranitidine concurrently (may need acid environment to work)

Adverse effects
Constipation
Diarrhoea
Hypophosphataemia

Cautions
Renal impairment (neurological adverse effects due to aluminium toxicity)
Risk of bezoar formation and potential intestinal obstruction
Interferes with absorption of quinolone antibiotics, phenytoin and digoxin when given orally

Organ failure
Renal: Aluminium may accumulate

Renal replacement therapy
No further dose modification is required during renal replacement therapy

*Used/standby
when
extubating*

SUXAMETHONIUM

The only depolarizing neuromuscular blocker available in the UK. It has a rapid onset of action (45–60 s) and a short duration of action (5 min). Breakdown is dependent on plasma pseudocholinesterase. It is best to keep the ampoule in the fridge to prevent a gradual loss of activity due to spontaneous hydrolysis.

Uses
Agent of choice for:

- rapid tracheal intubation as part of a rapid sequence induction

- for procedures requiring short periods of tracheal intubation, e.g. cardioversion

- management of severe post-extubation laryngospasm unresponsive to gentle positive pressure ventilation

Contraindications
History of malignant hyperpyrexia (potent trigger)
Hyperkalaemia (expect a further increase in K^+ level by 0.5–1.0 mmol/l)
Patients where exaggerated increase in K^+ (>1.0 mmol/l) are expected:

- severe burns

- extensive muscle damage

- disuse atrophy

- paraplegia and quadriplegia

- peripheral neuropathy, e.g. Guillain Barré

Administration
As a rapid sequence induction: 1.0–1.5 mg/kg IV bolus, after 3 min pre-oxygenation with 100% O_2 and a sleep dose of induction agent. Apply cricoid pressure until tracheal intubation confirmed. Intubation possible within 1 min. Effect normally lasting <5 min
Repeat dose of 0.25–0.5 mg/kg may be given. Atropine should be given at the same time to avoid bradycardia/asystole

How not to use suxamethonium
In the conscious patient
By persons not trained to intubate the trachea

Adverse effects
Malignant hyperpyrexia
Hyperkalaemia
Transient increase in IOP and ICP
Muscle pain
Myotonia
Bradycardia, especially after repeated dose

Cautions

Digoxin (may cause arrhythmias)
Myasthenia gravis (resistant to usual dose)
Penetrating eye injury ($\uparrow$ IOP may cause loss of globe contents)
Prolonged block in:

- patients taking aminoglycoside antibiotics, magnesium

- myasthenic syndrome

- pseudocholinesterase deficiency (inherited or acquired)

Organ failure

Hepatic: prolonged apnoea (reduced synthesis of pseudocholinesterase)

Given as a slow push down central line prior to new line being inserted.

TEICOPLANIN

This glycopeptide antibiotic, like vancomycin, has bactericidal activity against both aerobic and anaerobic Gram +ve bacteria: *Staphlococcus aureus*, including MRSA, *Streptococcus* spp., Listeria spp., and *Clostridium* spp. It is only bacteriostatic for most Enterococcus spp. It does not cause red man syndrome through histamine release and is less nephrotoxic than vancomycin. However due to variation in serum levels between patients effective therapeutic levels for severe infections may not be reached for a number of days using the most commonly recommended dosage schedules. Serum monitoring of pre-dose levels is recommended particularly for severe infections.

In the UK resistance is well recognised in enterococci and coagulase negative staphylococci and, more worryingly, is now emerging in *Staphylococcus aureus*.

Uses
Serious Gram +ve infections:

- prophylaxis and treatment of infective endocarditis (usually combined with gentamicin)
- dialysis-associated peritonitis
- infection caused by MRSA
- prosthetic device infections due to coagulase negative
- staphylococci
- alternative to penicillins and cephalosporins where patients are allergic

Contraindications
Hypersensitivity

Administration
IV bolus: 400 mg initially, then 200 mg daily. Give over 3–5 min.
For severe infections: 400 mg 12 hourly for 3 doses, then 400 mg daily.

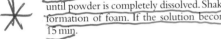Reconstitute with WFI supplied. Gently roll the vial between the hands until powder is completely dissolved. Shaking the solution will cause the formation of foam. If the solution becomes foamy allow to stand for 15 min.

Monitor: FBC, U&E, LFT
                  Serum pre dose teicoplanin level
Pre-dose (trough) serum concentration should not be <10 mg/l.
For severe infections, trough serum concentration >20 mg/l is recommended.

In renal impairment: dose reduction not necessary until day 4, then reduce dose as below:

CC (ml/min)	Dose*	Interval
40–60	1 unit dose	every 2 days
<40	1 unit dose	every 3 days

*Based on unit doses of 200 mg, 400 mg

How not to use teicoplanin
Do not mix teicoplanin and aminoglycosides in the same syringe

Adverse effects
Hypersensitivity
Blood disorders
Ototoxic
Nephrotoxic

Cautions
Vancomycin sensitivity
Renal/hepatic impairment
Concurrent use of ototoxic and nephrotoxic drugs

Organ failure
Renal: reduce dose

Renal replacement therapy
Removed by HF not HD (large molecule). Not removed by PD. For high clearance HF significance still only borderline, dose change not usually required. Can measure levels. Potential for low serum levels with high clearance systems, may need to dose as for 40–60 ml/min CC, particularly if high flux continuous haemofiltration is used.

TERLIPRESSIN

Oesophageal varices are enlarged blood vessels that form in the stomach or oesophagus as a complication of liver disease. When administered in bleeding oesophageal varices, terlipressin (*Glypressin*) is broken down to release lysine vasopressin, which causes vasoconstriction of these vessels thereby reducing the bleeding.

Uses
Bleeding oesophageal varices

Contraindications
Pregnancy

Administration
IV bolus: 2 mg, then 1–2 mg every 4–6 hourly, up to maximum of 3 days

Reconstitute with the supplied solvent containing sodium chloride and hydrochloric acid

Monitor: BP
             Serum sodium and potassium
             Fluid balance

Adverse effects
Abdominal cramps
Headache
Raised blood pressure

Cautions
Hypertension
Arrhythmias
Ischaemic heart disease

THIOPENTONE

Thiopentone is a barbiturate that is used widely as an IV anaesthetic agent. It also has cerebroprotective and anticonvulsant activities. Awakening from a bolus dose is rapid due to redistribution, but hepatic metabolism is slow and sedative effects may persist for 24 h. Repeated doses or infusion have a cumulative effect. Available in 500 mg ampoules or 2.5 g vial, which is dissolved in 20 or 100 ml WFI respectively to make a 2.5% solution.

Uses
Induction of anaesthesia
Status epilepticus (p. 208)

Contraindications
Airway obstruction
Previous hypersensitivity
Status asthmaticus
Porphyria

Administration
- IV bolus: 2.5–4 mg/kg. After injecting a test dose of 2 ml, if no pain, give the rest over 20–30 s until loss of eyelash reflex. Give further 50–100 mg if necessary

Reduce dose and inject more slowly in the elderly, patients with severe hepatic and renal impairment, and in hypovolaemic and shocked patients
In obese patients, dosage should be based on lean body mass

How not to use thiopentone
Do not inject into an artery (pain and ischaemic damage)
Do not inject solution >2.5% (thrombophlebitis)

Adverse effects
Hypersensitivity reactions (1:14 000–35 000)
Coughing, laryngospasm
Bronchospasm (histamine release)
Respiratory depression and apnoea
Hypotension, myocardial depression
Tachycardia, arrhythmias
Tissue necrosis from extravasation

Cautions
Hypovolaemia
Septic shock
Elderly (reduce dose)
Asthma

T

Organ failure
CNS: sedative effects increased
Cardiac: exaggerated hypotension and ↓ cardiac output
Respiratory: ↑ respiratory depression
Hepatic: enhanced and prolonged sedative effect. Can precipitate coma
Renal: increased cerebral sensitivity

TRANEXAMIC ACID

Tranexamic acid is an antifibrinolytic employed in blood conservation. It acts by inhibiting plasminogen activation.

Uses
Uncontrolled haemorrhage following prostatectomy or dental extraction in haemophiliacs
Haemorrhage due to thrombolytic therapy
Haemorrhage associated with DIC with predominant activation of fibrinolytic system

Contraindications
Thrombo-embolic disease
DIC with predominant activation of coagulation system

Administration
- Uncontrolled haemorrhage following prostatectomy or dental extraction in haemophiliacs

Slow IV: 500–1000 mg 8 hourly, given over 5–10 min (100 mg/min)

- Haemorrhage due to thrombolytic therapy

Slow IV: 10 mg/kg, given at 100 mg/min

- Haemorrhage associated with DIC with predominant activation of fibrinolytic system (prolonged PT, ↓ fibrinogen, ↑ fibrinogen degradation products)

Slow IV: 1000 mg over 10 min, single dose usually sufficient
Heparin should be instigated to prevent fibrin deposition

In renal impairment:

Serum creatinine (mmol/l)	Dose (mg/kg)	Interval
120–250	10	12 hourly
250–500	10	every 24 h
>500	5	every 24 h

How not to use tranexamic acid
Rapid IV bolus

Adverse effects
Dizziness on rapid IV injection
Hypotension on rapid IV injection

Cautions
Renal impairment (reduce dose)

Organ failure
Renal: reduce dose

Renal replacement therapy
No further dose modification is required during renal replacement therapy

VANCOMYCIN (Vancocin)

This glycopeptide antibiotic has bactericidal activity against aerobic and anaerobic gram +ve bacteria including MRSA. It is only bacteriostatic for most enterococci. It is used for therapy of *C. difficile* associated diarrhoea unresponsive to metronidazole, for which it has to be given by mouth. It is not significantly absorbed from the gut.

Serum level monitoring is required to ensure therapeutic levels are achieved and limit toxicity. Successful treatment of MRSA infections requires levels above the traditionally recommended range.

Vancomycin-resistant strains of enterococcus, (VRE), are well recognised in the UK. Resistance also occurs less commonly in coagulase negative staphylococci and is starting to emerge in rare isolates of S. aureus.

Uses
C. difficile associated diarrhoea via the oral route
Serious Gram +ve infections:

- prophylaxis and treatment of infective endocarditis (usually combined with gentamicin)

- dialysis-associated peritonitis

- infection caused by MRSA

- prosthetic device infections due to coagulase negative staphylococci

- alternative to penicillins and cephalosporins where patients are allergic

Contraindications
Hypersensitivity

Administration
- *C. difficile* associated diarrhoea

Orally: 125 mg 6 hrly for 7–10 days

- Infective endocarditis and other serious Gram +ve infections including those caused by MRSA

IV infusion: 500 mg 6 hourly, given over at least 60 min
or
1 g 12 hourly, given over at least 100 min
Duration of therapy is determined by severity of infection and clinical response. In staphylococcal endocarditis, treatment for at least 4 weeks is recommended. If pre-dose (trough) level is consistently less than 10 mg/l, decrease the dose interval to 8 hourly or 6 hourly. If the post-dose (peak) level is >30 mg/l, decrease the dose (see therapeutic drug monitoring page 194).

Vancomycin must be initially reconstituted by adding WFI:

- 250 mg vial – add 5 ml WFI
- 500 mg vial – add 10 ml WFI
- 1 g vial – add 20 ml WFI

The liquid in each reconstituted vial will contain 50 mg/ml vancomycin. Further dilution is required:

- Reconstituted 250 mg vial – dilute with at least 50 ml diluent
- Reconstituted 500 mg vial – dilute with at least 100 ml diluent
- Reconstituted 1 g vial – dilute with at least 200 ml diluent

Suitable diluent: 0.9% saline or 5% dextrose

Monitor: Renal function
           Serum vancomycin levels (p. 194)

How not to use vancomycin
Rapid IV infusion (severe hypotension, thrombophlebitis)
Not for IM administration

Adverse effects
Following IV use:

- Severe hypotension
- Flushing of upper body ('red man' syndrome)
- Ototoxic and nephrotoxic
- Blood disorders
- Hypersensitivity
- Rashes

Cautions
Concurrent use of:

- Aminoglycosides – ↑ ototoxicity and nephrotoxicity
- Loop diuretics – ↑ ototoxicity

Organ failure
Renal: reduce dose

Renal replacement therapy
Removed by HF not HD (large molecule 1468 daltons). Not removed by PD. For high flux HF, clearance significant. Levels must be monitored, and dose and interval adjusted accordingly. One gram can be given and a further dose when the trough level has fallen to 5–10 mg/l.

Dilute in 5% Dextrose

VASOPRESSIN

Vasopressin (antidiuretic hormone, ADH) controls water excretion in kidneys via V2 receptors and produces constriction of vascular smooth muscle via V1 receptors. In normal subjects vasopressin infusion has no effect on blood pressure but has been shown to significantly increase blood pressure in septic shock. The implication is that in septic shock there is a deficiency in endogenous vasopressin and this has been confirmed by direct measurement of endogenous vasopressin in patients with septic shock requiring vasopressors. In vitro studies show that catecholamines and vasopressin work synergistically.

Anecdotally, use of 3 units per hour is usually very effective and not associated with a reduction in urine output.

As its pseudonym antidiuretic hormone implies, vasopressin infusion might be expected to decrease urine output but the opposite is the case at doses required in septic shock. This may be due to an increase in blood pressure and therefore perfusion pressure. It is also worth noting that, whereas noradrenaline constricts the afferent renal arteriole, vasopressin does not, so may be beneficial in preserving renal function. It has been shown that doses as high as 0.1 units/minute (6 units/h) do reduce renal blood flow, so should be avoided. A dose of 0.04 units/min (2.4 units/hr) is often efficacious in septic shock and does not reduce renal blood flow.

Vasopressin does not cause vasoconstriction in the pulmonary or cerebral vessels, presumably due to an absence of vasopressin receptors. It does cause vasoconstriction in the splanchnic circulation, hence the use of vasopressin in bleeding oesophageal varices. The dose required in septic shock is much lower than that required for variceal bleeding.

Uses
In septic shock: reserve its use in cases where the noradrenaline dose exceeds 0.3 microgram/kg/min (unlicensed)

Contraindications
Vascular disease, especially coronary artery disease

Administration
IV infusion: 1–4 units/h
Dilute 20 units (1 ml ampoule of argipressin) in 20 ml 5% dextrose (1 unit/ml) and start at 1 unit/h, increasing to a maximum of 4 units/h

Do not stop the noradrenaline, as it works synergistically with vasopressin. As the patient's condition improves, the vasopressin should be weaned down and off before the noradrenaline is stopped.

Available as argipressin (*Pitressin*)
Stored in fridge between 2–8°C

VASOPRESSIN

How not to use vasopressin
Doses in excess of 5 units/h

Adverse effects
Abdominal cramps
Myocardial ischaemia
Peripheral ischaemia

Cautions
Heart failure
Hypertension

VECURONIUM

A non-depolarizing neuromuscular blocker with minimal cardiovascular effects. It is metabolized in the liver to inactive products and has a duration of action of 20–30 min. Dose may have to be reduced in hepatic/renal failure.

Uses
Muscle paralysis

Contraindications
Airway obstruction
To facilitate tracheal intubation in patients at risk of regurgitation

Administration
• Initial dose: 100 microgram/kg IV
• Incremental dose: 20–30 microgram/kg according to response

Monitor with peripheral nerve stimulator

How not to use vecuronium
As part of a rapid sequence induction
In the conscious patient
By persons not trained to intubate trachea

Cautions
Breathing circuit (disconnection)
Prolonged use (disuse muscle atrophy)

Organ failure
Hepatic: prolonged duration of action
Renal: prolonged duration of action

VERAPAMIL

A calcium channel blocker that prolongs the refractory period of the AV node.

Uses
SVT
AF
Atrial flutter

Contraindications
Sinus bradycardia
Heart block
Congestive cardiac failure
VT/VF – may produce severe hypotension or cardiac arrest
WPW syndrome

Administration
• IV bolus: 5–10 mg over 2 min, may repeat with 5 mg after 10 min if required

Continuous ECG and BP monitoring
Decrease dose in liver disease and in the elderly

How not to use verapamil
Do not use in combination with β-blockers (bradycardia, heart failure, heart block, asystole)

Adverse effects
Bradycardia
Hypotension
Heart block
Asystole

Cautions
Sick sinus syndrome
Hypertrophic obstructive cardiomyopathy
Increased risk of toxicity from theophylline and digoxin

Organ failure
Hepatic: reduce dose

VITAMIN K (Phytomenadione)

Vitamin K is necessary for the production of prothrombin, factors VII, IX and X. It is found primarily in leafy green vegetables and is additionally synthesized by bacteria that colonize the gut. Because it is fat-soluble, it requires bile salts for absorption from the gut. Patients with biliary obstruction or hepatic disease may become deficient. Vitamin K deficiency is not uncommon in hospitalized patients because of poor diet, parenteral nutrition, recent surgery, antibiotic therapy and uraemia.

Uses
Liver disease
Reversal of warfarin

Contraindications
Hypersensitivity
Reversal of warfarin when need for rewarfarinization likely (use FFP)

Administration
- Konakion® (0.5 ml ampoule containing 1 mg phytomenadione)

IV bolus: 1–10 mg, give over 3–5 min
Contains polyethoxylated castor oil which has been associated with anaphylaxis; should not be diluted

- Konakion® MM (1 ml ampoule containing 10 mg phytomenadione in a colloidal formulation)

IV bolus: 1–10 mg, give over 3–5 min
IV infusion: dilute with 55 ml 5% dextrose, give over 60 min. Solution should be freshly prepared and protected from light
Not for IM injection

Maximum dose: 40 mg in 24 h

How not to use vitamin K
Do not give by rapid IV bolus
Do not give IM injections in patients with abnormal clotting
Not for the reversal of heparin

Adverse effects
Hypersensitivity

Cautions
Onset of action slow (use FFP if rapid effect needed)

ZINC

Zinc is an essential constituent of many enzymes. Deficiencies in zinc may result in poor wound healing. Zinc deficiency can occur in patients on inadequate diets, in malabsorption, with increased catabolism due to trauma, burns and protein-losing conditions, and during TPN.

Hypoproteinaemia spuriously lowers plasma zinc levels.

Normal range: 12–23 μmol/l

Uses
Zinc deficiency
As an antioxidant (p. 222)

Administration
• Orally: Zinc sulphate effervescent tablet 125 mg dissolved in water, 1–3 times daily after food

Adverse effects
Abdominal pains
Dyspepsia

Voriconazole.

MIX with WFI
19ml / 200mg.

then reconstitute
with NaCl

Short
Notes

ROUTES OF ADMINISTRATION

Intravenous
This is the most common route employed in the critically ill. It is reliable, having no problems of absorption, avoids first-pass metabolism and has a rapid onset of action. Its disadvantages include the increased risk of serious side-effects and the possibility of phlebitis or tissue necrosis if extravasation occurs.

Intramuscular
The need for frequent painful injections, the presence of a coagulopathy (risk the development of a haematoma, which may become infected) and the lack of muscle bulk often seen in the critically ill means that this route is seldom used in the critically ill. Furthermore, variable absorption because of changes in cardiac output and blood flow to muscles, posture and site of injection makes absorption unpredictable.

Subcutaneous
Rarely used, except for heparin when used for prophylaxis against DVT. Absorption is variable and unreliable.

Oral
In the critically ill this route includes administrations via NG, NJ, PEG, PEJ or surgical jejunostomy feeding tubes. Medications given via these enteral feeding tubes should be liquid or finely crushed, dissolved in water. Rinsing should take place before and after feed or medication has been administered, using 20–30 ml WFI. In the seriously ill patient this route is not commonly used to give drugs. The effect of pain and its treatment with opioids, variations in splanchnic blood flow and changes in intestinal transit times as well as variability in hepatic function, make it an unpredictable and unreliable way of giving drugs.

Buccal and sublingual
Avoids the problem of oral absorption and first-pass metabolism, and it has a rapid onset time. It has been used for GTN, buprenorphine and nifedipine.

Rectal
Avoids the problems of oral absorption. Absorption may be variable and unpredictable. It depends on absorption from the rectum and from the anal canal. Drugs absorbed from the rectum (superior haemorrhoidal vein) are subject to hepatic metabolism; those from the anal canal enter the systemic circulation directly.

Tracheobronchial
Useful for drugs acting directly on the lungs: β_2-agonists, anticholinergics and corticosteroids. It offers the advantage of a rapid onset of action and a low risk of systemic side-effects.

LOADING DOSE

An initial loading dose is given quickly to increase the plasma concentration of a drug to the desired steady-state concentration. This is particularly important for drugs with long half-lives (amiodarone, digoxin). It normally takes five half-lives to reach steady-state if the usual doses are given at the recommended interval. Thus, steady-state may not be reached for many days. There are two points worth noting:

- For IV bolus administration, the plasma concentration of a drug after a loading dose can be considerably higher than that desired, resulting in toxicity, albeit transiently. This is important for drugs with a low therapeutic index (digoxin, theophylline). To prevent excessive drug concentrations, slow IV administration of these drugs is recommended.

- For drugs that are excreted by the kidneys unchanged (gentamicin, digoxin) reduction of the maintenance dose is needed to prevent accumulation. No reduction in the loading dose is needed.

DRUG METABOLISM

Most drugs are lipid-soluble and, therefore, cannot be excreted unchanged in the urine or bile. Water-soluble drugs such as the aminoglycosides and digoxin are excreted unchanged by the kidneys. The liver is the major site of drug metabolism. The main purpose of drug metabolism is to make the drug more water-soluble so that it can be excreted. Metabolism can be divided into two types:

- Phase 1 reactions are simple chemical reactions including oxidation, reduction, hydroxylation and acetylation.

- Phase 2 reactions are conjugations with glucuronide, sulphate or glycine. Many of the reactions are catalysed by groups of enzyme systems.

ENZYME SYSTEMS

These enzyme systems are capable of being induced or inhibited. Enzyme induction usually takes place over several days; induction of enzymes by a drug leads not only to an increase in its own metabolic degradation, but also often that of other drugs. This usually leads to a decrease in effect of the drug, unless the metabolite is active or toxic. Conversely, inhibition of the enzyme systems will lead to an increased effect. Inhibition of enzymes is quick, usually needing only one or two doses of the drug. Below are examples of enzyme inducers and inhibitors:

Inducers	Inhibitors
Barbiturates	Amiodarone
Carbamazepine	Cimetidine
Ethanol (chronic)	Ciprofloxacin
Inhalational anaesthetics	Dextropropoxyphene (co-proxamol)
Griseofulvin	Ethanol (acute)
Phenytoin	Etomidate
Primidone	Erythromycin
Rifampicin	Fluconazole
	Ketoconazole
	Metronidazole

DRUG EXCRETION

Almost all drugs and/or their metabolites (with the exception of the inhalational anaesthetics) are eventually eliminated from the body in urine or in bile. Compounds with a low molecular weight are excreted in the urine. By contrast, compounds with a high molecular weight are eliminated in the bile. This route plays an important part in the elimination of penicillins, pancuronium and vecuronium.

DRUG TOLERANCE

Tolerance to a drug will over time diminish its effectiveness. Tolerance to the effects of opioids is thought to be a result of a change in the receptors. Other receptors will become less sensitive with a reduction in their number over time when stimulated with large amounts of drug or endogenous agonist, for example catecholamines. Tolerance to the organic nitrates may be the result of the reduced metabolism of these drugs to the active molecule, nitric oxide, as a result of a depletion within blood vessels of compounds containing the sulphydryl group. Acetylcysteine, a sulphydryl group donor is occasionally used to prevent nitrate tolerance.

DRUG INTERACTIONS

Two or more drugs given at the same time may exert their effects independently or may interact. The potential for interaction increases the greater the number of drugs employed. Most patients admitted to an intensive care unit will be on more than one drug.

Drugs interactions can be grouped into three principal subdivisions: pharmacokinetic, pharmacodynamic and pharmaceutical.

- Pharmacokinetic interactions are those that include transport to and from the receptor site and consist of absorption, distribution, metabolism, and excretion.

- Pharmacodynamic interactions occur between drugs which have similar or antagonistic pharmacological effects or side-effects. This may be due to competition at receptor sites or can occur between drugs acting on the same physiological system. They are usually predictable from a knowledge of the pharmacology of the interacting drugs.

- Pharmaceutical interactions are physical and chemical incompatibilities may result in loss of potency, increase in toxicity or other adverse effect. The solutions may become opalescent or precipitation may occur, but in many instances there is no visual indication of incompatibility. Precipitation reactions may occur as a result of pH, concentration changes or 'salting-out' effects.

THERAPEUTIC DRUG MONITORING

The serum drug concentration should never be interpreted in isolation and the patient's clinical condition must be considered. The sample must be taken at the correct time in relation to dosage interval.

Phenytoin
Phenytoin has a low therapeutic index and a narrow target range. Although the average daily dose is 300 mg, the dose needed for a concentration in the target range varies from 100 to 700 mg/day. Because phenytoin has non-linear (zero order) kinetics, small increases in dose can result in greater increases in blood level.

Aminoglycosides
Gentamicin, tobramycin, netilmicin and amikacin are antibiotics with a low therapeutic index. After starting treatment, measurements should be made before and after the third to fifth dose in those with normal renal function and earlier in those with abnormal renal function. Levels should be repeated, if the dose requires adjustment, after another 2 doses. If renal function is stable and the dose correct, a further check should be made every 3 days, but more frequently in those patients whose renal function is changing rapidly. It is often necessary to adjust both the dose and the dose interval to ensure that both peak and trough concentrations remain within the target ranges. In spite of careful monitoring, the risk of toxicity increases with the duration of treatment and the concurrent use of loop diuretics.

Vancomycin
This glycopeptide antibiotic is highly ototoxic and nephrotoxic. Monitoring of serum concentrations is essential especially in presence of renal impairment.

Theophylline
Individual variation in theophylline metabolism is considerable and the drug has a low therapeutic index. Concurrent treatment with cimetidine, erythromycin and certain 4-quinolones (ciprofloxacin, enoxacin, norfloxacin) can result in toxicity due to enzyme inhibition of theophylline metabolism.

Digoxin
In the management of AF, the drug response (ventricular rate) can be assessed directly. Monitoring may be indicated if renal function should deteriorate and other drugs (amiodarone and verapamil) are used concurrently. The slow absorption and distribution of the drug means that the sample should be taken at least 6 h after the oral dose is given. For IV administration, sampling time is not critical.

TARGET RANGE OF CONCENTRATION

Drug	Sampling time(s) after dose	Threshold for therapeutic effect	Threshold for toxic effect
Teicoplanin	Trough: pre-dose	Trough: >10 mg/l Severe infections require >20mg/l	None defined
Gentamicin Tobramycin Netilmicin	Peak: 1 h after bolus or at end of infusion Trough: pre-dose	Peak: 10 mg/l	Trough: 2 mg/l
Vancomycin	Peak: 2 h after end of infusion Trough: pre-dose	Trough: 5–10 mg/l May need 15–20 mg/l for MRSA	Peak >30–40 mg/l
Phenytoin	Trough: pre-dose	None defined	20 mg/l (80 μmol/l)
Theophylline	Trough: pre-dose	10 mg/l (55 μmol/l)	20 mg/l (110 μmol/l)
Digoxin	At least 6 hrs	0.8 μg/l (1 nmol/l)	Dependent on plasma electrolytes, thyroid function, PaO_2

The target range lies between the lowest effective concentration and the highest safe concentration. Efficacy is best reflected by the peak level and safety (toxicity) is best reflected by the trough level (except for vancomycin). The dosage may be manipulated by altering the dosage interval or the dose or both. If the pre-dose value is greater than the trough, increasing the dosage interval is appropriate. If the post-dose value is greater than the peak, dose reduction would be appropriate.

PHARMACOLOGY IN THE CRITICALLY ILL

In the critically ill patient, changes of function in the liver, kidneys and other organs may result in alterations in drug effect and elimination. These changes may not be constant in the critically ill patient, but may improve or worsen as the patient's condition changes. In addition, these changes will affect not only the drugs themselves but also their metabolites, many of which may be active.

Hepatic disease

Hepatic disease may alter the response to drugs in several ways:

- Impairment of liver function slows elimination of drugs resulting in prolongation of action and accumulation of the drug or its metabolites.

- With hypoproteinaemia there is decreased protein binding of some drugs. This increases the amount of free (active) drug.

- Bilirubin competes with many drugs for the binding sites on serum albumin. This also increases the amount of free drug.

- Reduced hepatic synthesis of clotting factors increases the sensitivity to warfarin.

- Hepatic encephalopathy may be precipitated by all sedative drugs, opioids and diuretics that produce hypokalaemia (thiazides and loop diuretics).

- Fluid overload may be exacerbated by drugs that cause fluid retention, e.g. NSAID and corticosteroids.

- Renal function may be depressed. It follows that drugs having a major renal route of elimination may be affected in liver disease, because of the secondary development of functional renal impairment.

- Hepatotoxic drugs should be avoided.

Renal impairment

Impairment of renal function may result in failure to excrete a drug or its metabolites. The degree of renal impairment can be measured using creatinine clearance, which requires 24-h urine collection. It can be estimated by calculation using serum creatinine (see Appendix A). Serum creatinine depends on age, sex and muscle mass. The elderly patients and the critically ill may have creatinine clearances <50 ml/min but because of reduced muscle mass, increased serum creatinine may be 'normal'.

When the creatinine clearance is >30 ml/min, it is seldom necessary to modify normal doses, except for certain antibiotics and cardiovascular drugs which are excreted unchanged by the kidneys. There is no need to decrease the initial or loading dose. Maintenance doses are adjusted by either lengthening the interval between doses or by reducing the

size of individual doses or a combination of both. Therapeutic drug monitoring, when available, is an invaluable guide to therapy.

Haemofiltration or dialysis does not usually replace the normal excretory function of the kidneys. A reduction in dose may be needed.

Nephrotoxic drugs should, if possible, be avoided. These include frusemide, thiazides, sulphonamides, penicillins, aminoglycosides and rifampicin.

Cardiac failure
Drug absorption may be impaired because of GI mucosal congestion. Dosages of drugs that are mainly metabolized by the liver or mainly excreted by the kidneys may need to be modified. This is because of impaired drug delivery to the liver which delays metabolism and impaired renal function leading to delayed elimination.

CARDIOPULMONARY RESUSCITATION:

Adult Advanced Life Support Algorithm (The Resuscitation Council (UK) Guidelines 2005)

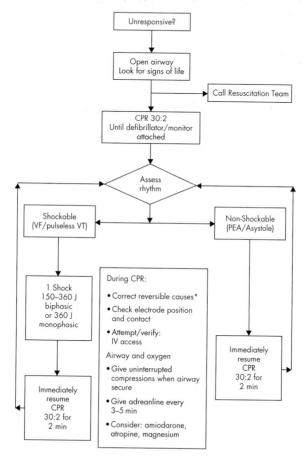

Unresponsive?

Open airway
Look for signs of life

Call Resuscitation Team

CPR 30:2
Until defibrillator/monitor attached

Assess rhythm

Shockable
(VF/pulseless VT)

Non-Shockable
(PEA/Asystole)

1 Shock
150–360 J
biphasic
or 360 J
monophasic

During CPR:

• Correct reversible causes*

• Check electrode position and contact

• Attempt/verify:
IV access

Airway and oxygen

• Give uninterrupted compressions when airway secure

• Give adrenaline every 3–5 min

• Consider: amiodarone, atropine, magnesium

Immediately
resume
CPR
30:2 for
2 min

Immediately
resume
CPR
30:2 for
2 min

*Reversible Causes

Hypoxia	Tension pneumothorax
Hypovolaemia	Tamponade (cardiac)
Hyper/hypokalaemia, hypocalcaemia &	Toxins
metabolic disorders	Thrombosis (coronary or pulmonary)
Hypothermia	

DRUGS IN ADVANCED LIFE SUPPORT

In VF/pulseless VT arrest, the administration of drugs should not delay DC shocks. Defibrillation is still the only intervention capable of restoring a spontaneous circulation. In EMD or PEA (pulseless electrical activity), the search for specific and correctable causes (4 Hs and 4 Ts) is of prime importance. If no evidence exists for any specific cause CPR should be continued with the use of adrenaline every 3–5 min.

Adrenaline (epinephrine) 1 mg (10 ml 1 in 10,000/ 1 ml 1 in 1,000)

Adrenaline has both alpha and beta effects. The alpha effect increases perfusion pressure and thus myocardial and cerebral blood flow. The beta-1 effect helps to maintain cardiac output after spontaneous heart action has been restored.

- VF/VT
Give adrenaline 1 mg IV if VF/VT persists after a second shock
Repeat adrenaline every 3–5 min if VF/VT persists

- PEA/asystole
Give adrenaline 1 mg IV as soon as IV access is achieved and repeat every 3–5 min

Amiodarone 300 mg IV

If VF/VT persists after 3 shocks, give amiodraone 300 mg as an IV bolus. A further 150 mg may be given for recurrent or refractory VF/VT, followed by an IV infusion of 900 mg over 24 h.

Lidocaine 1 mg/kg IV

If amiodarone is not available, lidocaine 1 mg/kg (7 ml of a 1% solution for a 70 kg individual) may be used as a second line drug. But do not give lidocaine if amiodarone has already been given.

Atropine 3 mg IV

For asystole and slow PEA (rate <60/min), immediately start CPR and give adrenaline 1 mg IV and atropine 3 mg IV as soon as IV access is achieved.
Atropine 3 mg will block vagal tone fully, so only one dose is recommended.

Magnesium 8 mmol IV (4 ml of a 50% solution)

Give magnesium 8 mmol for refractory VF if there is any suspicion of hypomagnesaemia (e.g. patients on potassium-losing diuretics). Other indications are:

- ventricular tachyarrhythmias in the presence of hypomagnesaemia
- torsade de pointes
- digoxin toxicity

Calcium chloride 1 g IV (10 ml of a 10% solution)

Adequate levels of ionised calcium are necessary for effective cardiovascular function. Ionised calcium concentrations decrease during prolonged (>7.5 min) cardiac arrest. The chloride salt is preferred to the gluconate salt, as it does not require hepatic metabolism to release the calcium ion. 10 ml 10% calcium chloride provides 6.8 mmol Ca^{2+} (10 ml 10% calcium gluconate provides only 2.25 mmol Ca^{2+}).

Caution: Calcium overload is thought to play an important role in ischaemic and reperfusion cell injury. It may also be implicated in coronary artery spasm. Excessive doses should not be used.

Calcium chloride is indicated in:

- Hypocalcaemia
- Hyperkalaemia
- calcium-channel antagonist overdose
- magnesium overdose

Sodium bicarbonate 50 mmol (50 ml of a 8.4% solution)

Routine use of sodium bicarbonate during cardiac arrest is not recommended.

Give 50 mmol of sodium bicarbonate if cardiac arrest is associated with hyperkalaemia or tricyclic antidepressant overdose. Repeat the dose according to the results of repeated blood gas analysis. Several problems are associated with its use:

(i) CO_2 released passes across the cell membrane and increases intracellular pH.
(ii) The development of an iatrogenic extracellular alkalosis may be even less favourable than acidosis.
(iii) It may induce hyperosmolarity causing a decrease in aortic diastolic pressure and therefore a decrease in coronary perfusion pressure.

Do not let sodium bicarbonate come into contact with catecholamines (inactivates) or calcium salts (precipitates).

Tracheobronchial route for drugs

If venous access is impossible, the tracheal route may be used for:

- adrenaline
- atropine
- lidocaine

Drug doses are 2–3 times that of the IV route. Dilute with 0.9% saline to a total of 10 ml and instilled deeply via a suction catheter or similar and give 5 large volume positive pressure breaths. Drug absorption may be impaired by atelectasis, pulmonary oedema, and – in the case of adrenaline – local vasoconstriction.

Do not give sodium bicarbonate and calcium chloride by this route.

MANAGEMENT OF ACUTE MAJOR ANAPHYLAXIS

- **Immediate therapy**
  Stop giving the suspect drug
  Maintain airway, give 100% oxygen
  Adrenaline 50–100 microgram (0.5–1.0 ml 1:10 000) IV
  Further 100 microgram bolus PRN for hypotension and bronchospasm
  Crystalloid 500–1000 ml rapidly

- **Secondary management**
  For adrenaline-resistant bronchospasm:
  salbutamol 250 microgram IV loading dose
  5–20 microgram/min maintenance
  dilute 5 mg in 500 ml 5% glucose or 0.9% saline (10 mcg/ml)
  or
  aminophylline 5 mg/kg
  in 500 ml 0.9% saline, IV infusion over 5 h
  To prevent further deterioration:
  hydrocortisone 200 mg IV
  and
  chlorphenamine 20 mg IV
  dilute with 10 ml 0.9% saline or WFI given over 1–2 min

- **Investigation**
  Plasma tryptase: Contact the Biochemistry lab first. Take 2 ml blood in an EDTA tube at the following times: as soon as possible (within 1 h), at 3 hours and at 24 hours (as control). The samples should be sent *immediately* to the lab for the plasma to be separated and frozen at −20 °C. When all the samples have been collected, they will be sent to: Department of Immunology, Northern General Hospital, Herries Road, Sheffield S5 7AU Telephone: 0114 2715552

  Assay for urinary methyl histamine is no longer available.

MANAGEMENT OF SEVERE HYPERKALAEMIA

Criteria for treatment:

- $K^+ > 6.5\,mmol/l$
- ECG changes (peaked T, wide QRS)
- Severe weakness

Calcium chloride 10–20 ml 10% IV over 5–10 min

This increases the cell depolarization threshold and reduces myocardial irritability. It results in improvement in ECG changes within seconds, but because the K^+ levels are not altered, the effect lasts only about 30 min.

Soluble insulin 10 units with 50 ml 50% glucose (50 g)

Given IV over 30–60 min. Begins lowering serum K^+ in 2–5 min and the effect lasting 1–2 h. Monitor blood glucose.

Sodium bicarbonate 50 mmol (50 ml 8.4%)

By correcting the acidosis its effect again is only transient. Beware in patients with fluid overload.

Calcium resonium 15 g PO or 30 g as retention enema, 8 hourly

This will draw the K^+ from the gut and remove K^+ from the body. Oral lactulose 20 ml 8 hourly may induce a mild diarrhoea, which helps to remove K^+ and also avoids constipation when resins are used.

Haemofiltration/dialysis

Indicated if: plasma K^+ persistently ↑; acidosis; uraemia; or when serious fluid overload is already present.

MANAGEMENT OF MALIGNANT HYPERTHERMIA

Clinical features
- Jaw spasm immediately after suxamethonium
- Generalized muscle rigidity
- Unexplained tachycardia, tachypnoea, sweating and cyanosis
- Increase in ETCO$_2$
- Rapid increase in body temperature ($>4°C/h$)

Management
- Inform surgical team and send for experienced help.
- Elective surgery: abandon procedure, monitor and treat.
- Emergency surgery: finish as soon as possible, switch to 'safe agents', monitor and treat.
- Stop all inhalational anaesthetics
- Change to vapour-free anaesthetic machine and hyperventilate with 100% O$_2$ at 2–3 times predicted minute volume.
- Give dantrolene 1 mg/kg IV.

  Response to dantrolene should begin to occur in minutes (decreased muscle tone, heart rate and temperature); if not, repeat every 5 min, up to a total of 10 mg/kg.
- Give sodium bicarbonate 100 ml 8.4% IV.

  Further doses guided by arterial blood gas.
- Correct hyperkalaemia with 50 ml 50% dextrose + 10 units insulin over 30 min.
- Correct cardiac arrhythmias according to their nature (usually respond to correction of acidosis, hypercarbia and hyperkalaemia).
- Start active cooling
  Refrigerated 0.9% saline IV 1–2 litres initially (avoid Hartmann's solution because of its potassium content).
  Surface cooling: ice packs and fans (may be ineffective due to peripheral vasoconstriction).
  Lavage of peritoneal and gastric cavities with refrigerated 0.9% saline.
- Maintain urine output with:
  IV fluids
  Mannitol
  Frusemide

Monitoring and investigations

ECG, BP and capnography (if not already).
Oesophageal or rectal temperature: core temperature.
Urinary catheter: send urine for myoglobin and measure urine output.
Arterial line: arterial gas analysis, U&E and creatine phosphokinase.
Central venous line: CVP and IV fluids.
Fluid balance chart: sweating loss to be accounted for.

After the crisis

Admit to ICU for at least 24 h (crisis can recur).
Monitor potassium, creatine phosphokinase, myoglobinuria, temperature, renal failure and clotting status.
May need to repeat dantrolene (half-life only 5 h).
Investigate patient and family for susceptibility.

Triggering agents

Suxamethonium
All potent inhalational anaesthetic agents

Safe drug

All benzodiazepines
Thiopentone, propofol
All non-depolarizing muscle relaxants
All opioids
Nitrous oxide
All local anaesthetic agents
Neostigmine, atropine, glycopyrrolate
Droperidol, metoclopramide

SEDATION, ANALGESIA AND NEUROMUSCULAR BLOCKADE

The ideal level of sedation should leave a patient lightly asleep but easily roused. Opioids, in combination with a benzodiazepine or propofol, are currently the most frequently used agents for sedation.

The most common indication for the therapeutic use of opioids is to provide analgesia. They are also able to elevate mood and suppress the cough reflex. This anti-tussive effect is a useful adjunct to their analgesic effects in patients who need to tolerate a tracheal tube.

Midazolam, the shortest acting of all the benzodiazepines is the most widely used. It can be given either by infusion or intermittent bolus doses.

Propofol has achieved widespread popularity for sedation, although it is expensive. It is easily titrated to achieve the desired level of sedation and its effects end rapidly when the infusion is stopped, even after several days of use. Propofol is ideal for short periods of sedation on the ICU, and during weaning when longer acting agents are being eliminated. Some clinicians recommend propofol for long-term sedation.

Currently new sedative and analgesic drugs are designed to be short-acting. This means that they usually have to be given by continuous IV infusion. The increased cost of these drugs may be justifiable if they give better control and more predictable analgesia and sedation, and allow quicker weaning from ventilatory support.

NSAID have an opioid-sparing effect and are of particular benefit for the relief of pain from bones and joints, as well as the general aches and pains associated with prolonged immobilization. However, their use in the critically ill is significantly limited by their side-effects, which include reduced platelet aggregation, gastrointestinal haemorrhage and deterioration in renal function.

Antidepressants may be useful in patients recovering from a prolonged period of critical illness. At this time depression and sleep disturbances are common. The use of amitriptyline is well established and relatively safe, but it has a higher incidence of antimuscarinic or cardiac side-effects than the newer agents. The beneficial effect may not be apparent until 2 weeks after starting the drug unless a large loading dose is given. Cardiovascular effects, in particular arrhythmias, have not proved to be a problem. Whether the newer SSRI (e.g. fluoxetine) will have any advantages in the critically ill remains to be proven.

Clomethiazole has sedative and anticonvulsant properties. It is usually reserved for patients with an alcohol problem.

Muscle relaxants are neither analgesic nor sedative agents and, therefore, should not be used without ensuring that the patient is both pain-free

and unaware. Their use has declined since the introduction of synchro-nized modes of ventilation and more sophisticated electronic control mechanisms. Suxamethonium, atracurium and vecuronium are presently the most commonly used agents, although pancuronium still retains a use in certain ICU. Their use should be restricted to certain specific indications:

- Tracheal intubation
- Facilitation of procedures, e.g. tracheostomy
- ARDS, where oxygenation is critical and there is risk of barotrauma
- Management of neurosurgical or head injured patients where coughing or straining on the tracheal tube increases ICP
- To stop the spasm of tetanus

Regular monitoring with a peripheral nerve stimulator is desirable; ablation of more than 3 twitches of the train-of-four is very rarely necessary.

SEDATION, ANALGESIA AND NEUROMUSCULAR BLOCKADE

SHORT NOTES

A PRACTICAL APPROACH TO SEDATION AND ANALGESIA

The way each ICU sedates its patients will depend on many factors. The number of doctors and nurses, design of the ICU (open plan versus single rooms) and the type of equipment are but some.

Midazolam and morphine given by IV boluses (2.5 mg) are a suitable regimen if a prolonged period of ventilatory support is anticipated and the patient does not have renal or hepatic impairment. An infusion can be started if this dose is required to be given frequently. Scoring of the level of sedation is essential. Once an infusion of either drug is started then its need should be reviewed on a daily basis and its dose reduced or stopped (preferably before the morning ward round) until the patient is seen to recover from the effects of the drug. Unnecessary use of infusions may induce tolerance. It should be remembered that although analgesics may provide sedation, sedatives do not provide analgesia; agitation caused by pain should be treated with an analgesic and not by increasing the dose of the sedative.

As the patient's condition improves and weaning from ventilatory support is anticipated, the morphine and midazolam can be stopped and an infusion of propofol and/or alfentanil started. This allows any prolonged effects of midazolam and morphine to wear off.

Such a regimen is effective both in terms of patient comfort and in avoiding the use of expensive drugs.

MANAGEMENT OF STATUS EPILEPTICUS

Status epilepticus is defined as continuous seizure activity lasting >30 min or more than two discrete seizures between which the patient does not recover consciousness. About 50% of patients have known epilepsy and status may be secondary to poor drug compliance with anticonvulsant therapy, a change in anticonvulsant therapy or alcohol withdrawal. Other causes of status epilepticus are listed below.

History of epilepsy

- Poor compliance
- Recent change in medication
- Drug interactions
- Withdrawal of the effects of alcohol
- Pseudostatus

No history of epilepsy

- Intracranial tumour/abscess
- Intracranial haemorrhage
- Stroke
- Head injury or surgery
- Infection – meningitis, encephalitis
- Febrile convulsions in children
- Metabolic abnormalities – hypoglycaemia, hypocalcaemia, hyponatraemia, hypomagnesaemia, hypoxia
- Drug toxicity
- Drug or alcohol withdrawal
- Use of antagonists in mixed drug overdoses

Status epilepticus is divided into four stages. There is usually a preceding period of increasing seizures – **the premonitory stage**, which can be treated with a benzodiazepine such as clobazam 10 mg. Early treatment at this stage may prevent the development of the next stage. **Early status epilepticus** can usually be terminated by an IV bolus of lorazepam 4 mg, repeated after 10 min if no response. If there is no response to benzodiazepine therapy after 30 min, **established status epilepticus** has developed and either phenobarbitone, phenytoin or fosphenytoin should be given. If a patient is in **refractory status epilepticus** (when seizure activity has lasted 1 h and there has been no response to prior therapy), the patient should be transferred to ICU and given a general anaesthetic to abolish electrographic seizure activity and prevent further cerebral damage.

The initial management of status epilepticus is directed at supporting vital functions. This is the same as that for any medical emergency, including assessment of airways, breathing and circulation.

IV **lorazepam** may now be the preferred first-line drug for stopping status epilepticus. Lorazepam carries a lower risk of cardiorespiratory depression (respiratory arrest, hypotension) than **diazepam** as it is less lipid-soluble. Lorazepam also has a longer duration of anticonvulsant activity compared with diazepam (6–12 h versus 15–30 min after a single bolus). If IV access cannot be obtained diazepam may be given rectally (Stesolid). It takes up to 10 min to work. The duration of action of diazepam in the brain is short (15–30 min) because of rapid redistribution. This means that although a diazepam bolus is effective at stopping a fit, it will not prevent further fits.

If there is no response to benzodiazepine treatment after 30 min, either **phenobarbitone**, **phenytoin** or **fosphenytoin** should be given. Fosphenytoin is a water-soluble phosphate ester of phenytoin that is converted rapidly after IV administration to phenytoin by endogenous phosphatases. An advantage of IV fosphenytoin is that it can be given up to three times faster than phenytoin without significant cardiovascular side-effects (hypotension, arrhythmias). It can also be given IM unlike phenytoin. Fosphenytoin may some day replace phenytoin. Patients with known epilepsy may already be on phenytoin. A lower loading dose should be given in these patients. Many of these patients will be having fits because of poor compliance. **Clomethiazole** is particularly useful where fits are due to alcohol withdrawal.

If the patient has not responded to prior therapy and seizure activity has lasted 1 h, the patient should be transferred to ICU and given a general anaesthetic (thiopentone or propofol) to abolish electrographic seizure activity and provide ventilatory support to prevent further cerebral damage. **Thiopentone** is a rapidly effective anticonvulsant in refractory status epilepticus and has cerebroprotective properties. Endotracheal intubation must be performed and the patient ventilated. Thiopentone has a number of pharmacokinetic disadvantages over propofol. Following an IV bolus, thiopentone is rapidly taken up in the brain, but high concentrations are not sustained due to its rapid redistribution into fatty tissues. For this reason an IV infusion should follow. Elimination of thiopentone may take days after prolonged infusion. Electroencephalographic monitoring is essential to ensure that the drug level is sufficient to maintain burst suppression. **Propofol** although not licensed for the treatment of status epilepticus has been used successfully. It certainly has pharmacokinetic advantages over thiopentone.

Paralysis with **suxamethonium**, **atracurium**, **vecuronium** or **pancuronium** is indicated if uncontrolled fitting causes difficulty in ventilation or results in severe lactic acidosis. Neuromuscular blockade should only be used in the presence of continuous EEG monitoring, as the clinical signs of seizure activity is abolished. Blind use of muscle relaxants without control of seizure activity may result in cerebral damage.

TREATMENT OF STATUS EPILEPTICUS

TREATMENT OF STATUS EPILEPTICUS

Initial measures
- **Position patient to avoid pulmonary aspiration of stomach contents**
- **Establish an airway (oropharyngeal or nasopharyngeal) and give 100% oxygen**
- **Monitor vital functions**
- **IV access**
- **Send bloods for FBC, U&E, calcium, glucose, anticonvulsant levels**
- **Arterial blood gas**

Lorazepam 4 mg IV
repeat after 10 mins if no response

If no response after 30 min

Phenobarbitone 10 mg/kg IV
given at a rate of 100 mg/min
or
Phenytoin 15 mg/kg IV
given at a rate of 50 mg/min
or
Fosphenytoin 15 mg/kg IV
given at a rate up to 150 mg/min

Monitor:
BP
ECG

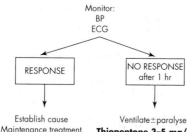

| RESPONSE | NO RESPONSE after 1 hr |

Establish cause
Maintenance treatment

Ventilate ± paralyse
Thiopentone 3–5 mg/kg IV
for intubation.
If continue to fit after 5 mins, give further
IV boluses of 50 mg PRN.
Then maintain on IV infusion at 50 mg/hr.
or
Propofol

Monitor: EEG

Further investigations after stabilisation
- **Serum magnesium**
- **LFTs**
- **CT±LP**
- **EEG**

REASONS FOR TREATMENT FAILURE

There are several possible reasons for failure of treatment, most of which are avoidable:

- Inadequate emergency anticonvulsant therapy
- Failure to initiate maintenance anticonvulsant therapy
- Metabolic disturbance, hypoxia
- Cardiorespiratory failure, hypotension
- Failure to identify or treat underlying cause
- Other medical complications
- Misdiagnosis (pseudostatus)

PSEUDOSTATUS

Up to 30% of patients ventilated for 'status epilepticus' may have pseudostatus. Clinical features suggestive of pseudostatus are:

- More common in females
- History of psychological disturbance
- Retained consciousness during 'fits'
- Normal pupillary response to light during 'fits'
- Normal tendon reflexes and plantar responses immediately after 'fits'

The diagnosis may be aided by EEG monitoring and serum prolactin level – raised following a true fit. A normal prolactin level is not helpful in that it does not exclude status epilepticus.

ANTI-ARRHYTHMIC DRUGS

The traditional Vaughan Williams' classification (based on electrophysiological action) does not include anti-arrhythmic drugs such as digoxin and atropine. A more clinically useful classification categorizes drugs according to the cardiac tissues which each affects, and may be of use when a choice is to be made to treat an arrhythmia arising from that part of the heart.

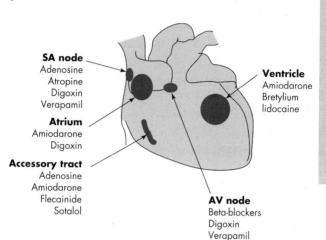

SA node
Adenosine
Atropine
Digoxin
Verapamil

Atrium
Amiodarone
Digoxin

Accessory tract
Adenosine
Amiodarone
Flecainide
Sotalol

Ventricle
Amiodarone
Bretylium
lidocaine

AV node
Beta-blockers
Digoxin
Verapamil

pamine, Dobutamine, Dopexamine, Adrenaline Noradrenaline

INOTROPES AND VASOPRESSORS

Inotropes: receptors stimulated

Drug	Dose (mcg/kg/min)	α_1	β_1	β_2	DA 1
Dopamine	1–5				+ +
	5–10		+	+	+ +
	>10	+	+	+	+ +
Dobutamine	1–25	0/+	+	+	
Dopexamine	0.5–6		0/+	+ + + +	+
Adrenaline	0.01–0.2	+/+ +	+	+	
Noradrenaline	0.01–0.2	+ + +	+		

Effects of inotropes

Drug	Cardiac contractility	Heart rate	SVR	Blood pressure	Renal and mesenteric blood flow
Dopamine: DA 1	0	0	0	0	+
β	+ +	+	0/+	+	0
α	0	0	+ +	+ +	−
Dobutamine	+ +	0	−	+	0
Dopexamine	0/+	+	−	0	+
Adrenaline	+ +	+	+/−	+	0/−
Noradrenaline	+	−	+ +	+ +	−

+, Increase; 0, no change; −, decrease

Which inotrope to choose?

The definition of a positive inotrope is an agent that will increase myocardial contractility by increasing the velocity and force of myocardial fibre shortening.

All inotropes will, therefore, increase myocardial oxygen consumption. In the case of a normal coronary circulation, the increased oxygen

Usually mixed with dextrose

demand caused by the increased inotropic state of the heart and the increase HR is met by increasing oxygen supply mediated by local mechanisms. In the presence of coronary artery disease, the increased oxygen demand may not be met by increase in coronary blood flow. The tachycardia shortens the coronary diastolic filling time reducing the coronary blood flow, making the ischaemia worse.

Therefore, inotropes have to be used with caution in patients with IHD.

The efficiency of the cardiac pump depends on preload, contractility, afterload and ventricular compliance. Each of these may be influenced by inotropes. In a patient with circulatory failure, an initial priority is to achieve an optimal preload by correcting any hypovolaemia. This may require the use of pulmonary artery catheter or oesophageal Doppler monitoring. If circulatory failure persists after optimal volume loading, a positive inotrope may be used to increase myocardial contractility. If intravascular volume has been restored (PCWP 10–15 mmHg) but perfusion is still inadequate, the selection should be based on the ability of the drug to correct or augment the haemodynamic deficit. If the problem is felt to be inadequate cardiac output, the drug chosen should have prominent activity at β_1 receptors and little α activity. If the perfusion deficit is caused by a marked reduction in SVR, then a drug with prominent α activity should be used. The haemodynamic picture is often more complex that those presented above. Other special considerations such as oliguria, underlying ischaemic heart disease or arrhythmias may exist and affect the choice of drug.

Most inotropes increase contractility by increasing the intracellular Ca^{2+} concentration of cardiac cells. This may be achieved in three different ways.

- The catecholamines stimulate the β_1 receptor, which activates adenyl cyclase resulting in increased cAMP. This causes opening of Ca^{2+} channels.

- PDE inhibitors prevent the breakdown of cAMP, thus facilitating Ca^{2+} entry and uptake by the sarcoplasmic reticulum.

- Digoxin acts by inhibiting Na^+/K^+ pump and increasing intracellular Ca^{2+} concentration indirectly through Na^+/Ca^{2+} exchange mechanism.

The other way to increase contractility is by increasing the sensitivity of the contractile protein, troponin C to Ca2+. Stretch and α adrenergic stimulation increase the sensitivity of troponin C for Ca2+.

Acidosis, hypoxia and ischaemia on the other hand, decrease the sensitivity of troponin C for Ca^{2+} and, therefore, the force of contraction.

There is no one ideal inotrope. The choice of inotrope will be influenced by the cause of the circulatory failure. The catecholamines are the most frequently used inotropes in the ICU. All act directly on adrenergic receptors. There are currently considered to be two α, two β

and five dopaminergic receptors. Adrenaline, noradrenaline and dopamine are naturally occurring catecholamines. Dopamine is the immediate precursor of noradrenaline, and noradrenaline is the precursor of adrenaline. Dobutamine is a synthetic analogue of isoprenaline that acts primarily on β receptors in the heart. Dopexamine is a synthetic analogue of dopamine, acting primarily on β_2 receptors.

Adrenaline (epinephrine) has α and β activities. In low dose, β predominates and SVR may be reduced. With high doses, α-mediated vasoconstriction predominates.

There is no stimulation of dopamine receptors. Adrenaline is useful when there is a severe reduction in cardiac output (e.g. cardiac arrest) in which the arrhythmogenecity and marked increase in HR and myocardial oxygen consumption that occur with this drug are not limiting factors. It is the drug of choice in anaphylactic shock, due to its activity at β_1 and β_2 receptors and its stabilizing effect on mast cells.

Noradrenaline (norepinephrine) is used to restore BP in cases of reduced SVR. The main haemodynamic effect of noradrenaline is predominantly α-mediated vasoconstriction. Noradrenaline can increase the inotropic state of the myocardium by α_1 and β_1 stimulation. The blood pressure is markedly increased due to vasoconstriction and the increase in myocardial contractility. However, cardiac output may increase or decrease due to the increase in afterload. The increase in blood pressure may cause reflex bradycardia. Noradrenaline will increase, PVR. It is a potent vasoconstrictor of the renal artery bed. It also produces vasoconstriction in the liver and splanchnic beds with reduced blood flow. But in septic shock, noradrenaline may increase renal blood flow and enhance urine production by increasing perfusion pressure. It can be used to good effect in septic shock when combined with dobutamine to optimize oxygen delivery and consumption. It is essential that the patient is adequately filled before starting noradrenaline. Indiscriminate use of noradrenaline can aggravate the oxygen debt because of peripheral vasoconstriction.

Dopamine exerts its haemodynamic effects in a dose-dependent way. In low doses it increases renal and mesenteric blood flow by stimulating dopamine receptors. The increase in renal blood flow results in increased GFR and increased renal sodium excretion. Doses between 2.5 and 10 mcg/kg/min stimulate β_1 receptors resulting in increased myocardial contractility, stroke volume and cardiac output. Doses >10 mcg/kg/min stimulate α receptors causing increased SVR, decreased renal blood flow and increased potential for arrhythmias. The distinction between dopamine's predominant dopaminergic and β effects at low doses and α effects at higher doses is not helpful in clinical practice due to marked interindividual variation. It may exert much of its effects by being converted to noradrenaline. However, because of overlap and individual variation, no dose is clearly only 'renal-dose' – dopaminergic effects may occur at higher doses, and vasoconstrictor effects at lower doses.

Dopamine tends to cause more tachycardia than dobutamine and unlike dobutamine usually increases rather than decreases pulmonary artery pressure and PCWP.

Dopamine has now been shown to have several adverse effects on other organ systems. On the respiratory system dopamine has been shown to reduce hypoxic respiratory drive and increase intra-pulmonary shunt leading to decreased oxygenation. Dopamine depresses anterior pituitary function except for ACTH secretion. Prolactin, LH, GH and thyroid hormones are all suppressed. This will obtund the body's acute endocrine response to stress.

Dopamine may also alter immunological function via its inhibitory effect on prolactin secretion. Inhibition of prolactin causes humoral and cell mediated immunosuppression.

With the current lack of evidence for renal protection and the numerous potential adverse effects, the use of dopamine for prevention of renal failure is highly questionable.

Dobutamine has predominant β_1 activity. It is used when the reduced cardiac output is considered the cause of the perfusion deficit, and should not be used as the sole agent if the decrease in output is accompanied by a significant decrease in BP. This is because dobutamine causes reductions in preload and afterload, which further reduce the BP. If hypotension is a problem, noradrenaline may need to be added.

Dopexamine is the synthetic analogue of dopamine. It has potent β_2 activity with one-third the potency of dopamine on the DA_1 receptor. There is no α activity. Dopexamine increases HR and CO, causes peripheral vasodilatation, $\uparrow$ renal and splanchnic blood flow, and $\downarrow$ PCWP. The current interest in dopexamine is centred on its dopaminergic and anti-inflammatory activity. The anti-inflammatory activity and improved splanchnic blood flow may be due to dopexamine's β_2 rather than DA 1 effect. Recent studies including one carried out in the ICU in York have shown reduced mortality in patients undergoing major surgery in those pre-optimized to a protocol which included pre-operative fluid and inotrope administration to achieve a target oxygen delivery. Our study suggests that dopexamine is superior to adrenaline when used in the pre-optimized protocol. This may be attributable to improved organ perfusion and oxygen delivery to organs such as the gut and the kidneys. In comparison with other inotropes, dopexamine causes less increase in myocardial oxygen consumption.

This synthetic agonist has a number of different properties but is mainly a β_2 agonist. Dopexamine acts as a positive inotrope to increase the heart rate and decrease the systemic vascular resistance. In animals, dopexamine increases renal blood flow by DA_1 agonism to cause intra-renal vasodilatation, an increased cortical but not medullary blood flow and an increase in urine output. However, in man the effects on diuresis and natriuresis are small, and may solely reflect the increase in renal

blood flow from the increased cardiac output. This results in an improved oxygen supply-demand balance compared with dopamine where the increased natriuresis is secondary to DA_2 activity, which increases oxygen requirements. Dopexamine also decreases gut permeability and may reduce bacterial translocation and endotoxinaemia.

There are two DA receptors with different functional activities (see table). Fenoldopam is a selective DA_1 agonist, introduced principally as an antihypertensive agent. It reduces blood pressure in a dose-dependent manner while preserving renal blood flow and GFR. As a DA_1 agonist, it acts postsynaptically to cause vasodilatation and so increase renal blood flow. Fenoldopam also improves creatinine clearance. It does not act as an inotrope, but is a selective vasodilator of both renal and mesenteric beds. Increasing doses of fenoldopam do not cause tachycardia or tachyarrhythmias, as the agent has no action on β or α receptors. However, a tachycardia may occur if there is rapid vasodilatation. It is not presently licensed in the UK. Use of fenoldopam was approved by the FDA for the treatment of accelerated hypertension in 1998; there has been increasing use of its renoprotective effects in doses ranging from 0.03 to 0.05 microgram/kg/min.

Table: Sites of action of dopaminergic receptor drugs and their agonist effects

Receptor	Site	Effects
DA_1	Renal and splanchnic beds	Vasodilatation, increased renal blood flow, natriuresis
DA_2	Postganglionic sympathetic nerves	Inhibits presynaptic norepinephrine release, decreases renal blood flow

Vasopressin

Vasopressin (antidiuretic hormone, ADH) controls water excretion in kidneys via V2 receptors and produces constriction of vascular smooth muscle via V1 receptors. In normal subjects vasopressin infusion has no effect on blood pressure but has been shown to significantly increase blood pressure in septic shock. The implication is that in septic shock there is a deficiency in endogenous vasopressin and this has been confirmed by direct measurement of endogenous vasopressin in patients with septic shock requiring vasopressors. In vitro studies show that catecholamines and vasopressin work synergistically. Anecdotally, use of 3 units/h is usually very effective and not associated with a reduction in urine output. As its pseudonym antidiuretic hormone implies, vasopressin infusion might be expected to decrease urine output but the opposite is the case at doses required in septic shock. This may be due to an increase in blood pressure and therefore perfusion pressure. It is also worth noting that, whereas noradrenaline constricts the afferent renal arteriole, vasopressin does not, so may be beneficial in preserving

renal function. It has been shown that doses as high as 0.1 units/minute (6 units/h) do reduce renal blood flow, so should be avoided. A dose of 0.04 units/min (2.4 units/hr) is often efficacious in septic shock and does not reduce renal blood flow. Vasopressin does not cause vasoconstriction in the pulmonary or cerebral vessels, presumably due to an absence of vasopressin receptors. It does cause vasoconstriction in the splanchnic circulation, hence the use of vasopressin in bleeding oesophageal varices. The dose required in septic shock is much lower than that required for variceal bleeding. It has been shown that doses as high as 0.1 units/minute (6 units/h) do reduce renal blood flow, so should be avoided. A dose of 0.04 units/min (2.4 units/h) is often efficacious and does not reduce renal blood flow. Anecdotally, use of 3 units/h is usually very effective and not associated with a reduction in urine output. In septic shock, its use is reserved for cases where the requirement for noradrenaline exceeds 0.3 mcg/kg/min. Vasopressin works synergistically with noradrenaline and as the patient's condition improves, the dose of vasopressin should be weaned down and off before the noradrenaline is stopped.

Enoximone and **milrinone** are both potent inodilators, and because they do not act via adrenergic receptors, they may be effective when catecholamines have failed. The inhibition of PDE III isoenzyme is responsible for the therapeutic effects. They can increase CO by 30–70% in patients with heart failure. They may also show synergy with catecholamines and have the added advantage of causing less ↑ myocardial oxygen consumption. Because they ↓ SVR and PVR, myocardial oxygen consumption is little increased compared with catecholamines. In addition they tend not to increase HR. There is also the added advantage of lusitropy – aiding relaxation of the ventricles and increasing coronary artery blood flow. The combination of inotropic support, vasodilatation, stable HR and improved diastolic relaxation is particularly advantageous in patients with IHD. Milrinone has an inotropy:vasodilatation ratio of 1:20 compared with 1:2 for enoximone. As a result, milrinone may need to be administered in combination with another inotrope or vasopressor.

The main use of enoximone and milrinone is the short-term treatment of severe congestive heart failure unresponsive to conventional therapy. In septic shock there is a significant risk of hypotension and they should be used with caution.

Digoxin has been used to treat heart failure for >200 years. The inotropic effect of digoxin is largely due to increase in intracellular calcium produced indirectly by inhibition of the Na/K pump. Its role in acute heart failure is restricted to patients in fast AF. In the presence of high sympathetic activity, its inotropic effect is negligible. It has a low therapeutic index. The potential for toxicity in the critically ill patient is increased by hypokalaemia, hypomagnesaemia, hypercalcaemia, hypoxia and acidosis. Toxicity does not correlate with plasma levels and is manifested by all types of arrhythmias, including AF.

BRONCHOSPASM

Causes of wheezing in the ICU

- Pre-existing asthma/COPD
- Anaphylactic reaction
- Aspiration pneumonia
- Kinked tracheal tube
- Tracheal tube too far – carinal/bronchial stimulation
- Bronchial secretions
- Pulmonary oedema
- Pneumothorax

Signs of severe asthma needing intensive care

- Tachycardia (HR > 130/min)
- Pulsus paradox > 20 mmHg
- Tachypnoea (RR > 30/min)
- Absent wheezing
- Exhaustion
- Inability to complete a sentence
- $PaCO_2$ normal or increased
- Hypoxia

The selective β_2 agonists such as salbutamol and terbutaline are the treatment of choice for episodes of reversible bronchospasm. Patients with chronic bronchitis and emphysema are often described as having irreversible airways obstruction, but they usually respond partially to the β_2 agonists or to the antimuscarinic drugs ipratropium or oxitropium. There is some evidence that patients who use β_2 agonists on a 'PRN' basis show greater improvement in their asthma than those using them on a regular basis. In the critically ill these drugs will have to be given either nebulized or intravenously. The tracheobronchial route is preferable because the drug is delivered directly to the bronchioles; smaller doses are then required, which cause fewer side-effects. If the bronchospasm is so severe that very little drug gets to the site of action via the tracheobronchial route, then the drug will have to be given IV.

ANTI-ULCER DRUGS

Critically ill patients are highly stressed and this leads to an increased incidence of peptic ulceration. The risk of stress ulceration is increased in the presence of:

- Sepsis
- Head injury
- Major surgical procedures
- Multiple trauma
- Severe burn injuries
- Respiratory failure
- Severe hepatic failure
- Severe renal failure

Routine use of anti-ulcer drugs to all patients in an ICU is unnecessary. Use should be restricted to those who have the risk factors described above and should be stopped when patients are established on enteral feeding.

IMMUNONUTRITION IN THE ICU

Patients admitted to the ICU may be malnourished at the time of admission, and certainly become so under the catabolic stress of major illness. The malnourished patient suffers from a reduction in immunity and is predisposed to infections. The importance of providing nutrition to critically ill patients is now widely accepted. Recently there has been a move to introduce certain dietary compounds with immune-enhancing actions to the feed. Compounds that have been found to have such properties include glutamine, arginine, nucleotides and omega–3 polyunsaturated fatty acids. None of these compounds when added into immune-enhancing enteral feeds have been shown to improve survival when compared with standard enteral feeds. However, most studies have shown reduction in infection rate, number of days ventilated and length of hospital stay. All these immune-enhancing formulas are significantly more expensive than standard formulas. In York, we supplement standard enteral feeds with glutamine (p. 94).

CORTICOSTEROIDS

While the normal physiological secretion of glucocorticoids from the adrenal cortex is about 30 mg cortisol per day, this can rise to 200–400 mg as part of the stress response to major surgery or trauma. Long-term therapy can suppress this adrenocortical response to stress. Patients on steroids or who have taken them within the past 12 months are also at risk of adrenal insufficiency. This may result in life-threatening hypotension, hyponatraemia and hyperkalaemia. The risk is greater when daily oral intake of prednisolone is >7.5 mg.

The aim in synthesizing new compounds has been to dissociate glucocorticoid and mineralocorticoid effects.

	Relative potencies		Equivalent dose (mg)
	Glucocorticoid	Mineralcorticoid	
Hydrocortisone	1	1	20
Prednisolone	4	0.25	5
Methylprednisolone	5	$\pm$	4
Dexamethasone	25	$\pm$	0.8
Fludrocortisone	10	300	–

In the critically ill patient, adrenocortical insufficiency should be considered when an inappropriate amount of inotropic support is required. Baseline cortisol levels and short synacthen test do not predict response to steroid. In patients who demonstrate a normal short synacthen test, yet show a dramatic response to steroid, it is possible that the abnormality lies in altered receptor function or glucocorticoid resistance rather than abnormality of the adrenal axis. Baseline cortisol levels and short synacthen test are worthwhile to assess hypothalamic-pituitary-adrenal axis dysfunction versus steroid unresponsiveness.

SHORT SYNACTHEN TEST

Before starting corticosteroid treatment, it is worth confirming the diagnosis of adrenal insufficiency. Failure of plasma cortisol to rise after IM/IV tetracosactrin 250 mcg indicates adrenocortical insufficiency.

Procedure:

- Contact lab first.
- Take 5 ml blood in a plain tube for cortisol before and 30 min after IM/IV tetracosactrin 250 mcg.

Interpretation:

- A normal response requires an incremental rise of at least 200 nmol/l and a final result must be >500 nmol/l. In the critically ill, values should be much higher. We normally accept 1000 nmol/l anywhere in the test as being a level sufficient for a septic patient needing ventilatory support.

The test is impossible to interpret once hydrocortisone has been started. If urgent treatment is required before test, use dexamethasone initially.

BONE MARROW RESCUE FOLLOWING NITROUS OXIDE

- Folic/folinic acid 15 mg IV for 2 days
- Vitamin B_{12} 1 mg IV for 2 days

The use of nitrous oxide for anaesthesia in excess of 2 h inactivates vitamin B_{12} and may lead to impaired DNA synthesis and megaloblastic bone marrow haemopoiesis. In fit patients this is of little significance, but in the critically ill it may increase the mortality rate. Haemopoeitic changes induced by nitrous oxide can be reversed by folic/folinic acid. Vitamin B_{12} is given to replace that which has been inactivated. It is recommended by some authorities that both folic/folinic acid and vitamin B_{12} should be given to critically ill patients following surgery in which nitrous oxide was used as part of the anaesthetic for >2 h.

ANTIOXIDANTS

The human body in health constantly produces potentially harmful reactive oxygen species. These are balanced by complex anti-oxidant systems. Tissue injury is probably due, at least in part, to local imbalances in the oxidant/anti-oxidant ratio. This imbalance is called 'oxidative stress' and can cause lipid peroxidation, damage to DNA and cell death. Sources of oxidative stress during critical illness include reactive oxygen species produced by leucocytes ('respiratory burst') and production of nitric oxide by vascular endothelium. Studies have suggested that the total anti-oxidant potential of the plasma is decreased in septic patients who go on to develop organ dysfunction.

A logical, if simplistic, approach to the oxidative stress of critical illness has been the administration of agents with free radical scavenging properties. The hope is that the oxidant/anti-oxidant ratio will be restored towards normal and tissue damage will, therefore, be reduced. Agents that have been used for this purpose include acetylcysteine, vitamins A, C and E, zinc and selenium. There remains no confirmed benefit and the use of such agents must be viewed as speculative.

- Acetylcysteine (p. 4)

- Zinc (p. 186)

- Vitamin C (ascorbic acid)
  orally: 1 g daily dispersible tablets
  slow IV: 1 g daily (500 mg/5 ml)

- Vitamin E (tocopheryl)
  orally: 100 mg 12 hourly (suspension 500 mg/5 ml)
  slow IV: 400 mg (oily injection 100 mg/2 ml)

- Selenium
  IV infusion: 400–800 mcg sodium selenite daily in 50 ml 0.9% saline, given over 1–4 h. Normal range: 70–120 μg/l. 0.88–1.52 μmol/l.

POST-SPLENECTOMY PROPHYLAXIS

Following splenectomy, patients have a lifelong increased risk of infection by encapsulated organisms such as *Strepococcus pneumoniae*, *Haemophilus influenzae* and *Neisseria meningitidis*. This is true whether the spleen was excised because of haematological malignancy or following trauma. Functionally asplenic patients (e.g. homozygous sickle cell disease) and those with congenital asplenia are similarly at risk.

Vaccinations and prophylactic antibiotics reduce but do not eliminate the risk of infection with these organisms.

Vaccinations

Vaccine	Dose	Repeat dose
Pneumovax II	0.5 ml by IM injection	Repeat every 5–10 years
Hiberix	0.5 ml by IM injection	No need
Meningitec or Menjugate	0.5 ml by IM or deep SC injection	No need

Annual influenza vaccine should be offered by the patient's GP.

Where possible the vaccines should be given 2 weeks before a splenectomy. Otherwise vaccination should optimally be given 2 weeks afterwards. This is because there is a dip in the immune response following major surgery. If it is not possible to organize this, a compromise is to vaccinate 3–5 days postoperatively (response suboptimal but adequate in most cases).

It is preferable for each vaccine to be given into different limbs.

The immunity conferred by the original meningococcal polysaccharide vaccine (Mengivac A + C) is not complete and is short-lived. Protection wanes rapidly and is generally gone by around 2 years from vaccination. The new conjugated meningococcal C vaccines are more effective and will provide long-term protection against infection by serogroup C of *Neisseria meningitidis*. Adults and any one aged under 25 years who has not been vaccinated previously with this vaccine should receive a single dose. This vaccine now forms part of the routine immunisation programme for a child. Group C infection accounts for around 40% of cases of meningococcal infection in the UK, most of the other cases are caused by group B infection, against which there is currently no vaccine.

However, when travelling to a high risk area for meningococcal infection, such patients will still require the additional protection conferred

by the polysaccharide A, C, W135 and Y tetravalent vaccine (*ACWY Vax*), even if they have already received meningococcal group C conjugate vaccine.

For individuals who have been given the meningococcal group C conjugate vaccine, an interval of at least 2 weeks should be allowed before giving the A, C, W135 and Y vaccine. For those patients who have already been vaccinated with the A, C, W135 and Y vaccine, an interval of at least 6 months should be allowed before the conjugated meningococcal C vaccine is given.

Antibiotic prophylaxis

Lifelong antibiotic prophylaxis should be offered to all patients.

Benzylpenicillin 600 mg 12 hourly IV or penicillin V 250 mg 12 hourly PO (omit if on cephalosporin prophylaxis for surgery).

If allergic to penicillin, erythromycin 500 mg 12 hourly IV or 250 mg 12 hourly PO.

ANTI-MICROBIAL DRUGS

Use of anti-microbial agents causes predictable adverse effects, which have to be considered as part of a risk/benefit analysis for each individual patient, the intensive care unit as a whole and for the wider hospital environment. These effects include superinfection, selection of resistant microorganisms and toxic side-effects. Close liaison with a clinical microbiologist is important to ensure correct use of these agents in order to minimise these effects.

Anti-microbial agents may be used in the following ways:

- Prophylactic – to prevent an infective complication
- Empiric – to treat suspected infection before culture results are available
- Targeted – to treat established infection demonstrated by culture

Infection is only one of a number of causes of pyrexia in the intensive care unit setting (see below). Administration of anti-microbial agents to all febrile patients is not appropriate and will lead to significant overuse of these agents, often with multiple changes of anti-microbial in a futile attempt to get the temperature to settle. A daily ward round with a clinical microbiologist or infectious disease physician can help to avoid this problem and provide an opportunity to evaluate the significance of new microbiological culture results. It is particularly worth bearing in mind the phenomenon of drug fever which is commonly caused by antibiotics and results in a pyrexia which only resolves when the provoking agent is discontinued.

Non-infective causes of pyrexia

SIRS Trauma Burns Pancreatitis Acute hepatic failure
Thrombotic events such as DVT and PE
Myocardial infarction
Fibroproliferative phase of ARDS
Drugs Antibiotics Hypnotics Diuretics Antihypertensives Antiarrhythmics NSAIDs

(Continued)

Non-infective causes of pyrexia (Continued)

Blood/blood product transfusion
Cancer Lymphoma Leukaemia Hypernephroma Hepatoma Pancreatic carcinoma
Connective tissue disease Systemic lupus erythematosus Polyarteritis nodosa Polymyalgia/cranial arteritis
Sarcoidosis
Rheumatoid disease
Malignant hyperpyrexia

Empiric therapy should be reserved for those patients with well defined signs and symptoms of infection where delay in therapy would be expected to be harmful. It is essential to obtain appropriate specimens for microbiological examination, before starting empiric therapy. Requests for rapid tests, such as Gram stains and antigen detection techniques, and invasive sampling techniques, such as broncho–alveolar lavage can be very helpful in guiding the need for empiric therapy and in modifying the choice of agents to be used.

The choice of agent(s) is also dependent on knowledge of the organisms likely to be involved. This should be based on previous experience within your own unit and should be designed to ensure coverage of the most likely pathogens, as failure to do so is associated with poorer patient outcomes. It should also take account of prior culture results for the individual patient concerned.

Anti-microbial therapy will not be successful in many infections associated with collections of pus or prosthetic devices without drainage or removal of the device as appropriate. Additional surgical intervention is not uncommonly required for intensive care unit patients.

Empiric therapy should be modified or stopped, as appropriate, once culture results become available. It is also good practice to have stop dates or review dates to avoid unnecessarily prolonged treatment or side-effects. Short course therapy of 5 to 7 days is adequate for most infections in the intensive care unit.

Although the majority of antibiotics are relatively safe drugs, important toxic effects do occur particularly in the presence of other disease states.

In addition, antibiotics may result in secondary bacterial, yeast or fungal infection (superinfection), and may facilitate the growth of *Clostridium difficile*, a cause of diarrhoea and pseudomembranous colitis.

Antibiotic resistance

Bacterial resistance to antibiotics is an established and increasing problem. Many pathogens are now 'multiresistant'. Excessive and inappropriate use of antibiotics is believed to be one of the most important factors in increasing the prevalence of antibiotic resistance. In most hospitals the intensive care unit has the highest prevalence of such organisms.

MRSA was first detected in Europe in the early 1960s. *Staphylococcus aureus* can survive for long periods in the environment and can colonise the skin, nose or throat of patients and health care staff. It is readily spread either via hands or by contact with the inanimate environment. In the UK, the prevalence of MRSA has been steadily rising. MRSA strains now account for up to 40% of all *Staphylococcus aureus* bloodstream infections in many hospitals in the UK. The majority of MRSA isolates in the UK belong to one of a relatively small number of epidemic strains (designated EMRSA), which have spread widely throughout the country. These strains usually express resistance to a number of antibiotics including macrolides, quinolones and beta-lactams. Traditionally, glycopeptides (vancomycin and teicoplanin) have been used to treat infections with these organisms although linezolid is now available as an alternative. Worryingly, glycopeptide resistance has now emerged in other parts of the world (notably Japan and the U.S.A).

MRSA is by no means the only bacterium in which the emergence of antibiotic resistance is a cause for concern. Cephalosporin-resistant Enterobacteriaceae (including *Klebsiella* spp., *E. coli* and *Enterobacter* spp.) expressing extended-spectrum beta-lactamases (ESBLs) are being identified with increasing frequency, and have caused outbreaks in hospitals and, more recently, in the community. As a result of growing problems with these organisms in the intensive care unit, empiric use of the carbapenems, imipenem and meropenem has increased. Unfortunately resistance to the carbapenems is well established in *Pseudomonas aeruginosa* isolates and is emerging in other Enterobacteriaceae and *Acinetobacter baumanii*.

Other problems include penicillin-resistant *Streptococcus pneumoniae*, which are being isolated from cases of community-acquired pneumonia, and quinolone resistant strains of *Salmonella typhi* and *paratyphi*, which are imported from the Indian sub-continent. Multidrug-resistant strains of *Mycobacterium tuberculosis* are still uncommon in the UK, but have caused outbreaks in two London hospitals.

Enterococci, which are inherently resistant to cephalosporins and fluroquinolones, have increasingly emerged as pathogens as the use of these drugs has increased. They are found in the stools of healthy people and can cause endogenous urinary tract and wound infections. *Enterococcus*

faecalis is the most frequent species to be cultured, but *Enterococcus faecium* has the greater inherent resistance. Beta-lactams alone are ineffective against most strains of *E. faecium*. It is especially worrying that resistance to glycopeptides is increasingly being reported from the US and the UK. Conventional treatments of serious enterococcal infections have involved the use of synergistic combinations of an aminoglycoside with a beta-lactam or a glycopeptide. *Enterococci* resistant to all synergistic combinations are now being reported.

Clostridium difficile infection

Clostridium difficile is a Gram +ve, spore-forming, toxin-producing, obligate anaerobic bacillus that is ubiquitous in nature. The increasing use of broad-spectrum antibiotics, sub-optimal infection control practice and the expanding population of patients with depressed immunity (renal, oncology, haematology and intensive care patients) have resulted in an increase in the frequency of outbreaks of infection, which may be prolonged and difficult to control. Since the first recognition of *C. difficile* infection in the late 1970s, reports have continued to escalate markedly. *C. difficile* has recently been labelled as a 'superbug' following outbreaks of a new virulent strain in the US, Canada, mainland Europe and in the UK that appears to be associated with poor outcome. Antibiotics particularly implicated are clindamycin, lincomycin and the cephalosporins (in particular 3rd generation), although any antibiotic can cause it, including those used to treat the infection (i.e. vancomycin and metronidazole). The most frequently implicated antibiotics causing *C. difficile* infection in the UK are amoxicillin and ampicillin, but this is probably a reflection of their high prescription rates. Patient presentation can range from asymptomatic colonization, diarrhoea (self-limiting through to severe diarrhoea due to pseudomembranous colitis), toxic megacolon, colonic perforation and death.

BACTERIAL GRAM STAINING

	Positive	Negative
COCCI	Enterococcus spp. Staphylococcus spp. Streptococcus spp. Streptococcus pneumoniae	Moraxella catarrhalis Neisseria spp.
RODS	Actinomyces israelii Clostridium spp. Corynebacterium diphtheriae Listeria monocytogenes	Bacteroides Burkholderia Enterobacter spp. Escherichia coli Haemophilus influenzae Klebsiella aergenes Legionella pneumophila Proteus mirabilis Pseudomonas aeruginosa Salmonellae Serratia marcescens Shigellae Stenotrophomonas

ANTIBIOTICS: SENSITIVITIES

	Ampicillin	Benzylpenicillin	Cefuroxime	Cefotaxime	Ceftazidime	Ceftriaxone	Ciprofloxacin	Co-amoxiclav	Erythromycin	Flucloxacillin	Gentamicin	Imipenem	Linezolid	Meropenem	Metronidazole	Tazocin	Teicoplanin	Vancomycin
S. aureus																		
MRSA																		
S. pyogenes																			
S. pneumoniae																			
E. faecalis																			
H. influenzae																			
E. coli																			
Klebsiella spp																			
N. meningitidis																			
P. mirabilis																			
Serratia spp																			
Ps. aeruginosa																			
B. fragilis																			
Clostridium spp																			

Legend:

- ■ Usually sensitive
- ▨ Many strains resistant
- □ Resistant or not recommended

When referring to this chart it is important to bear in mind the following:

- There is increasing antibiotic resistance in many organisms.

- There may be a great difference between antibiotic sensitivity determined *in vitro* and clinical use.

- There are great geographical variations in antibiotic sensitivity, not only between different countries, but also between different hospitals.

- Flucloxacillin may have activity against *S. pneumoniae,* but it is not used to treat pneumococcal pneumonia.

- *N. meningitidis* is not resistant to imipenem, but it would not be used for treatment because of neurotoxicity.

- *N. meningitidis* is not resistant to cefuroxime, although it would not be used for treatment of meningitis because of a high relapse rate.

RENAL REPLACEMENT THERAPY

Techniques available

Renal support in intensive care varies substantially between units. In the early days of intensive care, renal support was limited to either **haemodialysis** or **peritoneal dialysis**. Advances in membrane technology lead to the development of 'continuous arteriovenous haemofiltration' (CAVH). The driving pressure in this system is the patient's blood pressure; the blood is taken from an artery and returned to a vein. An ultrafiltrate of plasma water is produced, which is replaced by 'replacement fluid' that resembles plasma water but is devoid of the 'unwanted' molecules and ions, such as urea, creatinine and potassium. Fluid removal is achieved by replacing only a proportion of the volume of the fluid filtered. The development of CAVH enabled renal support to be undertaken on intensive care even in the absence of facilities for haemodialysis.

CAVH is now rarely used because of its problems, which include the dependence on systemic blood pressure, the need for large bore arterial access and, even when running optimally, poor clearances. Some of these problems have been at least partly overcome by the development of the now most commonly used renal replacement technique used in the critically ill, 'continuous veno-venous haemofiltration' (CVVH).

Peritoneal dialysis has limited use in critically ill patients. It is efficient at fluid removal but is inefficient in removal of toxic solutes and is often completely inadequate in the catabolic critically ill patient. Protein loss, hyperglycaemia, risk of infection and diaphragmatic splinting further contribute to its limited use in the critically ill.

In continuous veno-venous haemofiltration (**CVVH**) blood is removed and returned into large bore venous access by use of a mechanical pumping system. The higher blood flow rates achievable mean greater clearances, even in the presence of systemic hypotension, and the use of double-lumen central venous catheters has reduced the problems of vascular access. The simplicity of CAVH has been lost as the use of a mechanical pump has made necessary pressure monitors for the limbs of the vascular access, a bubble trap, and an air detector. Incorporated in modern systems are also systems for measuring the filtrate, adjusting and infusing the replacement fluid and infusing anticoagulants. A further refinement is the use of **haemodiafiltration** in which an element of dialysis is added to the clearance of solute by haemofiltration. In haemofiltration the membrane acts like a sieve in which plasma water is lost through the membrane pores, driven by the transmembrane pressure gradient. The membrane allows passage of molecules up to about 30 000 daltons molecular weight, although other factors such as charge and plasma protein binding will also affect clearance. In dialysis a dialysate is passed in the opposite direction to the flow of blood. The membrane used for dialysis is of smaller pore size than that used for haemofiltration and allows clearance of molecules up to about 500 daltons. In haemodiafiltration a haemofiltration membrane is used and a dialysate

fluid (often more haemofiltration replacement fluid) is pumped countercurrent to the blood flow through the filtrate space. The filtrate and dialysate fluid are collected together. The use of the dialysate particularly increases the clearance of the lower molecular weight molecules, such as urea (60 daltons) and creatinine (113 daltons).

Early reports of haemodialysis described marked haemodynamic instability in critically ill patients with its use and this contributed to the predominance of haemofiltration in the renal support of the critically ill. More recent reports demonstrate a reduction in haemodynamic instability with the use of modern membranes and techniques. The exact technique used for renal support in the critically ill depends on local policy and availability.

There is continuing interest, in the ability of haemofiltration to remove so-called 'middle molecules'. These are molecules that are too large to be cleared by conventional haemodialysis, but are demonstrably cleared by haemofiltration. These include molecules such as TNF α (molecular weight 16 500 daltons). Whether the removal of these molecules with high flow haemofiltration reaches clinically significant levels of clearance and leads to clinical benefit remains controversial.

Haemofiltration membranes are made of synthetic polymers such as polysulfone or polyacrylonitrile. These are supplied as a cylindrical canister in which there are several thousand hollow fibres held within a plastic casing. The blood passes down the middle of the hollow fibres with filtrate emerging into the space between the fibres.

Composition of haemofiltration replacement fluid:

Sodium	140 mmol/l
Chloride	115 mmol/l
Calcium	1.75 mmol/l
Magnesium	0.75
Sodium lactate	3.36 g/l
Dextrose	1 g/l
Potassium	nil (may need to be added)
Phosphate	nil
Osmolarity	293 mosm/l

Composition of lactate-free replacement fluid:

Sodium	110 mmol/l
Chloride	115 mmol/l
Calcium	1.75 mmol/l
Magnesium	0.75

In exceptional circumstances, lactate-free haemodiafiltration with systemic IV infusion of sodium bicarbonate may be needed in severe liver disease or lactic acidosis. The sodium bicarbonate cannot be added to the replacement fluid as this will result in an unstable solution. Failure to infuse sodium bicarbonate will result in severe hyponatraemia and worsening acidosis, as the patient's own bicarbonate is filtered out. The

sodium bicarbonate requirement is 30 mmol per litre of replacement fluid or 750 mmol per 25-litre exchange. Remember that 1 ml 8.4% sodium bicarbonate solution is equivalent to 1 mmol sodium and 1 mmol bicarbonate.

Creatinine clearances

The clearances achieved by renal replacement therapies are very variable, but roughly are in the region of:

Technique	Creatinine clearance
CAVH	9 ml per min
CVVH	15 ml per min
CVVHD	25–40 ml per min
IHD	160 ml per min
PD	3 ml per min

CVVHD = continuous veno-venous haemodiafiltration
IHD = intermittent haemodialysis
PD = peritoneal dialysis

The much higher clearances with haemodialysis allow intermittent treatment. Some units use a large haemofilter with high flow rates and achieve much higher clearances which allows intermittent haemofiltration. Adequate clearances can be achieved with lower performance techniques if used continuously.

RENAL REPLACEMENT THERAPY

SHORT NOTES

EXTRACORPOREAL DRUG CLEARANCE: BASIC PRINCIPLES

- Extracorporeal elimination is only likely to be significant if its contribution to total body clearance exceeds 25–30%
- Neither renal failure nor renal replacement therapy requires adjustment of the loading dose. This depends on the volume of distribution.
- The maintenance doses of drugs that are normally substantially cleared by the kidneys should be adapted to the effective clearance of the replacement therapy of the particular drug.
- Extracorporeal elimination only replaces glomerular filtration (i.e. no tubular secretion or reabsorption). As a consequence there are potential inaccuracies in using the creatinine clearance of a replacement therapy as a basis of drug dosage calculation.
- If the volume of distribution is large changes in tissue concentration due to extracorporeal elimination will be small
- Only free drug in plasma can be removed
- Other factors affecting clearance include:
- the molecular weight of the drug
- the lipid solubility of the drug
- the permeability and binding characteristics of the membrane
- the actual technique employed (such as dialysis or filtration)
- For haemofiltration it is customary to refer to the 'sieving coefficient'.

$$\text{Sieving coefficient (S)} = \frac{\text{concentration in ultrafiltrate}}{\text{concentration in plasma}}$$

For urea and creatinine the sieving coefficient $= 1$

Elimination of drugs by any extracorporeal system will vary according to the details of the technique used, such as the membrane surface area, blood flow rate, duration of cycle.

The clearance of any drug by pure haemofiltration (clearance by 'convection' Cl_{HDF}) is, therefore, obtained by multiplying the sieving coefficient by the ultrafiltration rate (Q_F volume of filtration per unit time):

$$Cl_{HDF} = S \times Q_F$$

DRUG DOSES IN RENAL FAILURE/RENAL REPLACEMENT THERAPY

It is convenient to divide drugs into four groups:

- Those requiring no dose reduction in renal failure.
- Those that may require a dose reduction in renal failure.
- Those requiring no further dose modification during renal replacement therapy.
- Those that may require further dose modification due to renal replacement therapy.

Drugs requiring NO DOSE MODIFICATION in renal failure

Acetylcysteine	Heparin
Adenosine	Hydrocortisone
Adrenaline	Insulin
Alfentanil	Isoprenaline
Amiodarone	Ipratropium
Amitryptiline	Labetolol
Atracurium	Lactulose
Atropine	Lignocaine
Calcium	Loperamide
Ceftriaxone	Methylprednisolone
Chlormethiazole	Naloxone
Cyclizine	Nifedpine
Cyclosporin	Nimodipine
Dalteparin	Noradrenaline
Desmopressin	Nystatin
Dexamethasone	Ondanetron
Dobutamine	Phentolamine
Dopamine	Phenytoin
Dopexamine	Propofol
Doxapram	Protamine
Epoprostenol	Salbutamol
Epoietin	Suxamethonium
Esmolol	Thiopentone
Fentanyl	Vecuronium
Flumazenil	Verapamil
Glutamine	Vitamin K
Glycerol suppository	Zinc
Granisetron	

Drugs that MAY REQUIRE A DOSE MODIFICATION in renal failure

Aciclovir	Haloperidol
Amphotericin	Hydralazine
Ampicillin	Imipenem/Cilastatin
Benzylpenicillin	Magnesium sulphate
Bumetanide	Mannitol
Captopril	Meropenem
Ceftazidime	Metoclopramide
Cefuroxime	Midazolam
Ciprofloxacin	Milrinone
Co-amoxiclav	Morphine
Codeine phosphate	Pancuronium
Co-trimoxazole	Pentamidine
Diazepam	Pethidine
Diclofenac	Phenobarbitone
Digoxin	Phosphate supplements
Droperidol	Pipericillin/tazobactam
Enalapril	Potassium supplements
Enoximone	Prochlorperazine
Erythromycin	Pyridostigmine
Flucloxacillin	Ranitidine
Fluconazole	Sucralfate
Frusemide	Teicoplanin
Ganciclovir	Tranexamic acid
Gentamicin	Vancomycin

Drugs requiring NO FURTHER DOSE MODIFICATION during renal replacement therapy

Aminophylline	Imipenem/Cilastatin
Amphotericin	Mannitol
Bumetanide	Metoclopramide
Captopril	Metronidazole
Cefotaxime	Midazolam
Ciprofloxacin	Milrinone
Codeine phosphate	Pancuronium
Diazepam	Pentamidine
Diclofenac	Pethidine
Droperidol	Phenobarbitone
Enalapril	Pipericillin/tazobactam
Enoximone	Prochlorperazine
Erythromycin	Pyridostigmine
Flucloxacillin	Ranitidine
Frusemide	Sucralfate
Haloperidol	Tranexamic acid
Hydralazine	

Drugs that MAY REQUIRE DOSE MODIFICATION during renal replacement therapy

Aciclovir – removed by HD and HF, similar to urea clearance. Elimination will only be significant for high clearance systems. Dose as for CC 10–25 ml/min. Not significantly cleared by PD.

Ampicillin – removed by HD/HF/PD but significant only for high clearance technique. Dose as for CC 10–20 ml/min.

Benzylpenicillin – removed by HD/HF/PD but significant only for high clearance techniques. Dose as for CC 10–20 ml/min (75% dose).

Ceftazidime – removed by HD/HF/PD, significant for high clearance techniques when suggested dose is 1g daily in divided doses. For low clearance techniques dose as for CC <10 ml/min. Levels can be monitored. If high clearance technique dose as for CC 10–20 ml/min.

Cefuroxime – removed by HD/HF/PD but significant only for high clearance techniques. Dose for high clearance renal replacement 750 mg 12 hourly. For low clearance techniques dose as for CC <10 ml/min.

Co-amoxiclav – removed by HD/HF/PD but significant only for high clearance techniques. Dose as for CC 10–20 ml/min. Pharmacokinetics of the amoxycillin and clauvulanate are closely matched, probably cleared at similar rates.

Co-trimoxazole – removed by HD/HF but significant only with high clearance techniques. Give 30 mg twice a day (or 60 mg once a day) if low clearance technique or 60 mg twice a day for 3 days followed by 30 mg twice a day (or 60 mg once a day) if high clearance technique. Plasma levels of sulphamethoxazole and trimethoprim can be measured and are useful in renal failure and support. Not significantly removed by PD.

Digoxin – removed by HD/HF but significant only with high clearance techniques. Dose according to measured plasma levels. With high clearance levels likely dose needed 125–250 mcg per day, 62.5 mcg per day or less with low clearance technique. Not significantly removed by PD.

Fluconazole – removed by HD/HF/PD but significant only for high clearance technique. For high clearance technique dose as in normal renal function, halve dose if low clearance. For intermittent renal therapy give half dose after each treatment.

Ganciclovir – the major route of clearance of ganciclovir is by glomerular filtration of the unchanged drug. Removed by HD and HF similar to urea clearance, only likely to be significant for high clearance systems. Dose on the basis of the achieved serum creatinine. For intermittent renal therapy give dose after treatment. Clearance by PD not likely to achieve clinical significance.

Gentamicin – removed by HD/HF/PD. Levels must be monitored, and dose and interval adjusted accordingly. Dose according to achieved creatinine clearance. For intermittent therapy give after treatment.

Magnesium sulphate – removed by HD/HF/PD. Accumulates in renal failure, monitor levels.

Meropenem – removed by HD and probably by HF. For high clearance techniques it is probably sensible to dose as for CC 10–25 ml/min. Clearance by PD not likely to achieve clinical significance.

Morphine – removed by HD/HF but significant only with high clearance techniques – also removes active metabolite morphine 6-glucuronide which accumulates in renal failure. Titrate to response. Not significantly removed by PD.

Phosphate supplements – phosphate accumulates in renal failure. Removed by HD/HF but significant only with high clearance techniques. Treat hypophosphataemia only on the basis of measured serum levels.

Potassium supplements – potassium accumulates in renal failure. Removed by HD/HF/PD. Treat hypokalaemia only on the basis of measured serum levels.

Teicoplanin – removed by HF not HD (large molecule). Not removed by PD. For high clearance HF significance still only borderline, dose change not usually required. Can measure levels. Potential for low serum levels with high clearance systems, may need to dose as for 40–60 ml/min CC, particularly if high flux continuous haemofiltration is used.

Vancomycin – removed by HF not HD (large molecule of 1468 daltons). Not removed by PD. For high flux HF, clearance significant. Levels must be monitored, and dose and interval adjusted accordingly. 1 g can be given and a further dose when the trough level has fallen to 5–10 mg/l.

CHEMICAL PLEURODESIS OF MALIGNANT PLEURAL EFFUSION

Until recently, tetracycline was the most widely used but is now no longer available worldwide. Doxycycline and talc are now the 2 recommended sclerosing agents. They are thought to work by causing inflammation of the pleural membranes. This procedure can be painful. In the awake patient, administer between 15–25 ml lidocaine 1% (maximum dose 3 mg/kg) via the chest drain immediately prior to the sclerosing agent. Intravenous opioids and paracetamol may be required. Anti-inflammatory drugs, such as NSAIDs and steroids should be avoided for up to two days before and after the procedure if possible. Talc has a high success rate and is usually well tolerated. Pleuritic chest pain and mild fever are the commonest side effects. However, ARDS is associated with the use of talc in less than 1% of cases. Doxycycline has no serious complications and tends to be the first choice with talc reserved for recurrent effusions. The major disadvantages of bleomycin are the cost and the need for trained personnel familiar with the handling of cytotoxic drugs.

Procedure:
- Ensure drainage of the effusion and lung re-expansion
- Analgesics in the awake patient
- Clamp drain at patient's end and insert 50 ml bladder syringe filled with 3 mg/kg lidocaine (20 ml 1% solution for 70 kg patient)
- Release clamp and inject the lidocaine slowly into the pleural space
- Clamp drain and in the same manner inject either doxycycline 500 mg or talc 2 to 5 g or bleomycin 60,000 units (4 vials) diluted in up to 50 ml 0.9% saline with the bladder syringe
- Flush drain with 10 ml 0.9% saline
- Clamp the drain for 60 min, observing for signs of increasing pneumothorax (tachycardia, hypotension, falling oxygen saturation, decrease tidal volumes)
- When talc is used, encourage patient to roll onto both sides if possible
- Unclamp the drain and leave on free drainage
- In the absence of excessive fluid drainage (>250 ml/day), the drain should be removed within 3 days of sclerosant administration
- If excessive fluid drainage persists (>250 ml/day), repeat pleurodesis with alternative sclerosant

Sclerosing agent	Dose	Success rate	Side effects	Cost
Doxycycline	500 mg	76%	Chest pain (40%), fever	£23
Talc	2 to 5 g	90%	Chest pain (7%), fever, ARDS (<1%)	4 g £11
Bleomycin	60,000 units	61%	Chest pain, fever, nausea	£65

Reference: British Thoracic Society Guidelines for the management of malignant pleural effusions. *Thorax* 2003; **58** (suppl II); ii29–ii38.

Appendices

APPENDIX A: CREATININE CLEARANCE

Severity of renal impairment is expressed in terms of glomerular filtration rate, usually measured by creatinine clearance. Creatinine clearance may be estimated from the serum creatinine.

Estimating creatinine clearance from serum creatinine:

For men:

$$\text{CC (ml/min)} = \frac{\text{weight (kg)} \times (140\text{-age}) \times 1.23}{\text{serum creatinine } (\mu\text{mol/L})}$$

For women:

$$\text{CC (ml/min)} = \frac{\text{weight (kg)} \times (140\text{-age}) \times 1.03}{\text{serum creatinine } (\mu\text{mol/L})}$$

Normal range (Based on an adult with a body surface area of $1.73\,\text{m}^2$):

Age	Sex	CC (ml/min)
20–29	Male	94–140
	Female	72–110
30–39	Male	59–137
	Female	71–121

For each decade thereafter values decrease by 6.5 ml/min.

Renal impairment is arbitrarily divided into three grades:

Grade	CC (ml/min)
Mild	20–50
Moderate	10–20
Severe	<10

Renal function declines with age; many elderly patients have a glomerular filtration rate <50 ml/min, which, because of reduced muscle mass, may not be indicated by a raised serum creatinine. It is wise to assume at least mild renal impairment when prescribing for the elderly.

APPENDIX B: WEIGHT CONVERSION (STONES/LB TO KG)

		lb						
	0	**2**	**4**	**6**	**8**	**10**	**12**	**13**
6	38.1	39.0	40.0	40.8	41.7	42.6	43.5	44.0
7	44.5	45.4	46.3	47.2	48.1	49.0	49.9	50.3
8	50.8	51.7	52.6	53.5	54.4	55.3	56.2	56.7
9	57.2	58.1	59.0	59.9	60.8	61.7	62.6	63.0
10	63.5	64.4	65.3	66.2	67.1	68.0	68.9	69.4
11	69.9	70.8	71.7	72.6	73.5	74.4	75.4	75.7
12	76.2	77.1	78.0	78.9	79.8	80.7	81.6	82.1
13	82.6	83.5	84.4	85.3	86.2	87.0	88.0	88.4
14	88.9	89.8	90.7	91.6	92.5	93.4	94.3	94.8
15	95.3	96.2	97.1	98.0	98.9	99.8	100.7	101.1
16	101.6	102.5	103.4	104.3	105.2	106.1	107.0	107.5
17	108.0	108.9	109.8	110.7	111.6	112.5	113.4	113.8
18	114.3	115.2	116.1	117.0	117.9	118.8	119.7	120.2

(Row labels 6–18 under **STONES**)

APPENDIX C: BODY MASS INDEX (BMI) CALCULATOR

$$BMI = \frac{Height\ (in\ metres)^2}{Weight\ (kg)}$$

To use the table:

First convert weight to kg (1 lb = 0.45 kg).

Then read across from patient's height until you reach the weight nearest to the patient's.

Then read up the chart to obtain the BMI.

Height Feet/ inches	Metres	20	21	22	23	24	25	26	27	28	29	30
5'0"	1.52	46	49	51	53	55	58	60	62	65	67	69
5'1"	1.55	48	50	53	55	58	60	62	65	67	70	72
5'2"	1.58	50	52	55	57	60	62	65	67	70	72	75
5'3"	1.60	51	54	56	59	61	64	67	69	72	74	77
5'4"	1.63	53	56	58	61	64	66	69	72	74	77	80
5'5"	1.65	54	57	60	63	65	68	71	74	76	79	82
5'6"	1.68	56	59	62	65	68	71	73	76	79	82	85
5'7"	1.70	58	61	64	66	69	72	75	78	81	84	87
5'8"	1.73	60	63	66	69	72	75	78	81	84	87	90
5'9"	1.75	61	64	67	70	74	77	80	83	86	89	92
5'10"	1.78	63	67	70	73	76	79	82	86	89	92	95
5'11"	1.80	65	68	71	75	78	81	84	87	91	94	97
6'0"	1.83	67	70	74	77	80	84	87	90	94	97	100
6'1"	1.85	68	72	75	79	82	86	89	92	96	99	103
6'2"	1.88	71	74	78	81	85	88	92	95	99	102	106
6'3"	1.90	72	76	79	83	87	90	94	97	101	105	108
6'4"	1.93	74	78	82	86	89	93	97	101	104	108	112
6'5"	1.96	77	80	84	88	92	96	99	103	107	111	115
		Desirable						Moderately obese				

<20 = underweight

20 to 24.9 = desirable

25 to 29.9 = moderately obese

>30 = obese

APPENDIX D: LEAN BODY WEIGHT CHARTS

For men:

Height in feet & inches (cm)	Weight (kg)		
	Small Frame	Medium Frame	Large Frame
5'6" (168 cm)	62–65	63–69	66–75
5'7" (170 cm)	63–66	65–70	68–76
5'8" (173 cm)	64–67	66–71	69–78
5'9" (175 cm)	65–68	69–74	70–80
5'10" (178 cm)	65–70	69–74	72–82
5'11" (180 cm)	66–71	70–75	73–84
6'0" (183 cm)	68–73	71–77	75–85
6'1" (185 cm)	69–75	73–79	76–87
6'2" (188 cm)	70–76	75–81	78–90
6'3" (191 cm)	72–78	76–83	80–92
6'4" (193 cm)	74–80	78–85	82–94

For women:

Height in feet & inches (cm)	Weight (kg)		
	Small Frame	Medium Frame	Large Frame
5'0" (152 cm)	47–52	51–57	55–62
5'1" (155 cm)	48–54	52–59	57–64
5'2" (158 cm)	49–55	54–60	58–65
5'3" (160 cm)	50–56	55–61	60–67
5'4" (163 cm)	52–58	56–63	61–69
5'5" (165 cm)	53–59	58–64	62–70
5'6" (168 cm)	55–60	59–65	64–72
5'7" (170 cm)	56–62	60–67	65–74
5'8" (173 cm)	57–63	62–68	66–76
5'9" (175 cm)	59–65	63–70	68–77
5'10" (178 cm)	60–66	65–71	69–79
5'11" (180 cm)	61–67	66–72	70–80
6'0" (183 cm)	63–69	67–74	72–81

APPENDIX E: INFUSION RATE/ DOSE CALCULATION

To calculate the infusion rate in ml/h:

$$\text{Infusion rate (ml/hr)} = \frac{\text{Dose (mcg/kg/min)} \times \text{Weight (kg)} \times 60}{\text{Concentration of solution (mcg/ml)}}$$

• To calculate the dose in mcg/kg/min:

$$\text{Dose (mcg/kg/min)} = \frac{\text{Infusion rate (ml/hr)} \times \text{Concentration of solution (mcg/ml)}}{\text{Weight (kg)} \times 60}$$

For example: Adrenaline infusion (4 mg made up to 50 ml) running at 6 ml/hr in a patient weighing 80 kg.

$$\text{Dose (mcg/kg/min)} = \frac{6 \text{ ml/hr} \times \dfrac{400 \text{ mcg}}{50 \text{ ml}}}{80 \text{ kg} \times 60}$$

$$= 0.1 \text{ mcg/kg/min}$$

APPENDIX F: DRUG COMPATIBILITY CHART

Ideally, all drugs given intravenously should be given via a dedicated line or lumen, and not mixed at any stage. However, if this is not possible, then compatibility data must be obtained before co-administering drugs. In general, drugs should not be added to parenteral nutrition. Blood products, sodium bicarbonate and mannitol should not be used for intravenous drug administration.

As a general guide, line compatibility of different drugs often depends on the pH of the drugs concerned. This will vary depending on how the drug is reconstituted or diluted. Drugs with widely differing pH will almost certainly be incompatible. However, the converse is not necessarily true, and lines should always be checked regularly for any gross signs of incompatibility (e.g. precipitate formation).

This chart indicates whether two drugs can be run in through the same IV access. It assumes normal concentrations and infusion rates for each drug, and data may vary depending on the diluent used. It should be used as a guide only, and not taken as definitive.

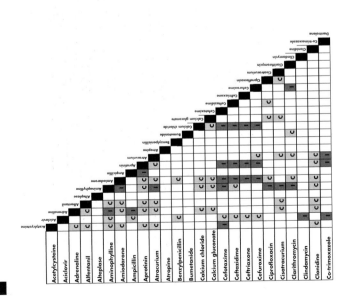

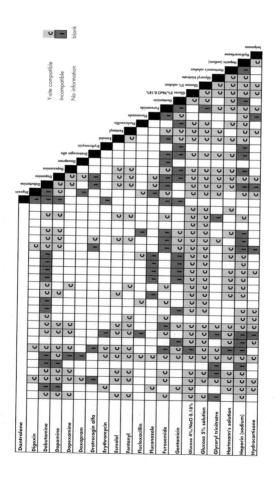

APPENDIX F: DRUG COMPATIBILITY CHART

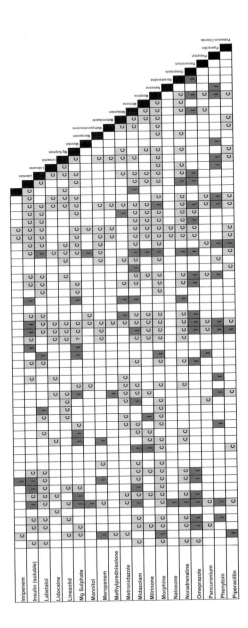

																																																																		Potassium Phosphate	Propofol	Ranitidine	Remifentanil	Salbutamol	Sodium bicarbonate	Sodium Chloride 0.9%	Streptokinase	Thiopental	Tranexamic Acid	Vancomycin	Vasopressin	Verapamil
Potassium Chloride		C	C			C	C	C		C	C	C		C	C		C			C	C	C				I	C	C	C	C	C	C		C	C		C	C		C	C		C	C			C	C	C	C	C	I		I		C	C	C		C			I	C														
Potassium Phosphate														I	I					I								I				I		C														C			C																												
Propofol		C	C	C		C		I	I	I	I		C	I	I	C	C	C	C	I	I					I	I	C	C	C				C	C	I	C	C	I	C	C	C	C	C	C	C	C	C	C		I	C		I		C	C	C		C		I	I	I	C														
Ranitidine		C				C				C	C					C	C	C	C	C		C						C	C						C	C	C	C		C	C			C				C		C								C		C		C		C			I												
Remifentanil	C		C	C		C	C		C	C										C	C			C				C	C	C				C	C				C	C	C	C	C	C			C	C			C	C			C	C		C		C	I				C		C											
Salbutamol						I																																C		C	C							C										C									I											
Sodium Bicarbonate				I		C	I							I	I	I	I			I	I							I	I	I	I			I			C			C	C		I	C			C	I	I		I	C				I	C	I	I	I		I			C	I	C		C									
Sodium chloride 0.9%	C	C	C	C		C	I	C	C	C		C	C	C	C	C	C	C	C	C	C	C	C	C	C		C	C	C	C		C	C	C	C	C		C	C	C	C	C	C	C			C	C			C	C	C	C	C	C	C	C	C	C	C		C	C	C		C	C	C	C	C							
Streptokinase							C							C													C													C	C			C					C																														
Thiopental			I	I		I				I	I										I							I	I	I			C	I	C			I		C	C	C	I	C			I	I	I							I	C	I		I					C		C		C		I							
Tranexamic Acid																																	I							C	C		C	C																														C						
Vancomycin		C				C	C			C					C	I	I	I	I		C	C										I		C			C			C	C		C	I			C	C		C	C					C	C	C				C			C		C		C		I	C						
Vasopressin			C				C																					C	C			I									C	C		C													C			C												C						
Verapamil							C	I												C		C					C	C	C																					C																	I											

APPENDIX G: OMEPRAZOLE ADMINISTRATION RECORD

York Hospitals **NHS**

NHS Trust

Prescription chart for omeprazole infusion

This regimen gives an omeprazole dose of 80 mg iv over 1 hour (given as 2 × 40 mg each over 30 minutes), then a continuous infusion of 8 mg/hr for 72 hours.

Notes:
- Ensure you have the correct omeprazole preparation i.e. infusion NOT injection
- Omeprazole vial is compatible with a 100 ml minibag plus of sodium chloride 0.9%

ENTER KNOWN DRUG ALLERGIES/ SENSITIVITIES OR WRITE NIL KNOWN		First Name:
		Surname:
		D.O.B.:
		Hosp. No.:
Dr's Signature: N.B. PATIENT MUST HAVE RED ALLERGY BAND IN SITU	Bleep:	Consultant
		Weight

Date	Route	Infusion fluid	Volume	Additions to Infusion		Time to run or ml/hour	Prescriber's signature	Batch no.	Actual start time & date	Signature		Asset no. of pump: (if used)
				Drug	Dose					Administered by	Checked by	
	IV	Sodium chloride 0.9%	100 ml	Omeprazole	40 mg	30 min (200 ml/h)						
	IV	Sodium chloride 0.9%	100 ml	Omeprazole	40 mg	30 min (200 ml/h)						
	IV	Sodium chloride 0.9%	100 ml	Omeprazole	40 mg	5 h (20 ml/h)						

(Continued)

IV	Sodium chloride 0.9%	100 ml	Omeprazole	40 mg	5 h (20 ml/h)		
IV	Sodium chloride 0.9%	100 ml	Omeprazole	40 mg	5 h (20 ml/h)		
IV	Sodium chloride 0.9%	100 ml	Omeprazole	40 mg	5 h (20 ml/h)		
IV	Sodium chloride 0.9%	100 ml	Omeprazole	40 mg	5 h (20 ml/h)		
IV	Sodium chloride 0.9%	100 ml	Omeprazole	40 mg	5 h (20 ml/h)		
IV	Sodium chloride 0.9%	100 ml	Omeprazole	40 mg	5 h (20 ml/h)		
IV	Sodium chloride 0.9%	100 ml	Omeprazole	40 mg	5 h (20 ml/h)		
IV	Sodium chloride 0.9%	100 ml	Omeprazole	40 mg	5 h (20 ml/h)		
IV	Sodium chloride 0.9%	100 ml	Omeprazole	40 mg	5 h (20 ml/h)		
IV	Sodium chloride 0.9%	100 ml	Omeprazole	40 mg	5 h (20 ml/h)		
IV	Sodium chloride 0.9%	100 ml	Omeprazole	40 mg	5 h (20 ml/h)		
IV	Sodium chloride 0.9%	100 ml	Omeprazole	40 mg	5 h (20 ml/h)		
IV	Sodium chloride 0.9%	100 ml	Omeprazole	40 mg	5 h (20 ml/h)		
IV	Sodium chloride 0.9%	100 ml	Omeprazole	40 mg	5 h (20 ml/h)		

APPENDIX H: DROTRECOGIN PRESCRIBING CRITERIA

York Hospitals **NHS**

NHS Trust

Prescribing criteria checklist for drotrecogin alfa (activated)

Affix addressograph label

Patient name
Address

DOB   Hosp No.

Indication for use: Adult patients with severe sepsis and more than one organ failure.

Inclusion criteria:	
Less than 48 hours after the onset of the first sepsis induced organ dysfunction.	If yes, continue. If no, stop here.
Patient is receiving optimum intensive care support?	If yes, continue. If no, stop here.
Patient has known or suspected infection defined as: ❏ Positive culture ❏ Leucocytes in a normally sterile body fluid ❏ Perforated viscus ❏ Radiological and clinical evidence of pneumonia (X-ray/purulent sputum) ❏ Other syndrome with high probability of infection (e.g., ascending cholangitis)	1 or more? If yes, continue. If no, patient not eligible.
Patient has three or more signs of SIRS defined as: ❏ Core temp of $\geq 38°C$ or $\leq 36°C$ ❏ HR of ≥ 90 beats/min ❏ RR ≥ 20 breaths/min or $PaCO_2$ ≤ 4.3 kPa or mechanical ventilation for acute (not chronic) respiratory process ❏ WBC $\geq 12 \times 10^9/l$ or $\leq 4 \times 10^9/l$	3 or more? If yes, continue. If no, patient not eligible.
Dysfunction of two organs or systems defined as: ❏ CARDIOVASCULAR: Arterial systolic BP ≤ 90 mmHg or a mean arterial pressure (MAP) ≤ 70 mmHg for at least 1 hour	

(Continued)

despite adequate fluid resuscitation or adequate intravascular volume status **OR** The need for vasopressors to maintain systolic blood pressure (SBP) ≥90 mmHg or MAP ≥0 mmHg ❑ RENAL: Urine output <0.5 ml/kg/hr for >1 hour, despite adequate fluid resuscitation ❑ RESPIRATORY: PaO_2/FiO_2 <33 kPa if other dysfunctional organs; <27 if lung only affected organ ❑ HAEMATOLOGIC: Platelet count <80 × 10^9/l or decreased by 50% from highest value in the previous 72 hours **AND** Other evidence of DIC ❑ METABOLIC: Unexplained metabolic acidosis Base Excess more negative than −5.	2 or more? If yes, continue. If no, patient not eligible.

Exclusion criteria:

Contra-indications ❑ Age <18 years ❑ Active internal bleeding ❑ Patients with intracranial pathology; neoplasm or evidence of cerebral herniation ❑ Concurrent heparin therapy ≥15 international units/kg/hour ❑ Known bleeding diathesis except for acute coagulopathy related to sepsis ❑ Chronic severe hepatic disease including cirrhosis or varices or chronic jaundice ❑ Platelet count <30 × 10^9/l, even if platelet count is increased after transfusions ❑ Any surgery that requires general or spinal anaesthesia in the 12-hour period immediately preceding the drug infusion ❑ Any post-operative patient with evidence of active bleeding ❑ Any patient with planned or anticipated surgery during the drug infusion period (see administration guidelines) ❑ History of severe head trauma requiring hospitalization, intracranial or intraspinal surgery, or haemorrhagic stroke within the previous 3 months	1 or more? If no, continue. If yes, patient not eligible.

(Continued)

❑ History of intracerebral arteriovenous malformation, cerebral aneurysm or CNS neoplasm ❑ Presence of an epidural catheter during the infusion or within 6 hours of removal ❑ Gastro-intestinal bleeding within the last 6 weeks that has required medical intervention unless definitive surgery has been performed ❑ Trauma patients at increased risk of bleeding ❑ Known hypersensitivity to drotrecogin alfa (activated) or any component of the product ❑ Patient/family do not want to pursue aggressive medical care	

Cautions
❑ Weight >135 kg
❑ INR >3.0 or prothrombin time >36 seconds
❑ Recent (within 3 months) ischaemic stroke
❑ Recent administration (within 12 hours) of greater than 10,000 units of antithrombin III
❑ Patients who are pregnant or breastfeeding
❑ HIV positive with $<50 \times 10^6/l$ CD_4 cells
❑ Bone marrow, lung, liver, pancreas or small bowel transplant recipient
❑ Chronic renal failure requiring haemodialysis or peritoneal dialysis (acute renal failure is not an exclusion)
❑ Acute pancreatitis and no established source of infection
❑ Anticoagulation (any of those listed below)
  – Unfractionated heparin to treat active thrombotic event within 8 hours
  – Oral anticoagulants within 7 days
  – Low molecular weight heparin (dalteparin or enoxaparin) at a higher dose than recommended for prophylactic use within 12 hours of infusion
  – Clopidogrel; aspirin >650 mg/day; glycoprotein IIb/IIIa inhibitors
  – Thrombolytic therapy within 3 days
❑ Patient not expected to survive >28 days (moribund)
❑ Advanced stage cancer (end stage disease)
	1 or more?
	If no, continue.
	If yes, additional consideration required.

Patient meets all inclusion criteria and has no contra-indications	If yes, patient eligible.

ICU Consultant approval.................................... Date.....................

APPENDIX I: DROTRECOGIN ADMINISTRATION

York Hospitals **NHS**
NHS Trust

ADMINISTRATION OF DROTRECOGIN ALFA (activated)

Drotrecogin alfa (activated) (Activated Protein C, Xigris™) is a novel drug with anti-inflammatory, anticoagulant and pro-fibrinolytic properties. It has been shown to reduce mortality in septic patients, particularly in patients with multi-organ failure (defined by NICE as 2 or more major organs) when added to best standard care.

It is a very expensive drug and the Prescribing Criteria Checklist must be signed by the ICU Consultant to ensure the patient is eligible to receive drotrecogin alfa (activated) before the drug is made up and administered.

5 mg vial = £152   Treatment for an 80 kg patient will cost > £6000.

Dosage
- All patients should receive drotrecogin alfa (activated) at a dose of 24 microgram/kg/hour (use actual body weight) for up to 96 hours (4 days) by intravenous infusion.
- If the infusion is interrupted for any reason, Xigris should be restarted at the 24 microgram/kg/hour infusion rate and continued to complete the full recommended 96 hours of dosing administration.
- No dosage adjustment is required in acute renal or hepatic failure.

Prescription
Should state: Drotrecogin alfa (activated) 24 microgram/kg/hour for 96 hours xx kg

Preparation and Administration
- Drotrecogin alfa (activated) vials must be kept in the fridge
- Once reconstituted drotrecogin alfa (activated) is stable for up to 14 hours at room temperature so infusions must not run for longer than this
- Giving sets should be labelled with the time and date when the infusion was first started and changed every 48 hours
- Drotrecogin alfa (activated) should be administered via a dedicated intravenous line or a dedicated lumen of a multi-lumen central venous catheter
- See next page for reconstitution guidelines and administration rates based on patients weight.

Cautions and Adverse Events

The most likely adverse event with drotrecogin alfa (activated) is serious bleeding. The risk can be minimised by adhering to the recommended exclusion criteria (see Summary of Product Characteristics or Prescribing Criteria Checklist). If sequential measures of coagulopathy (including platelet count) indicate worsening or severe coagulopathy, the risk of continuing the infusion should be weighed against the expected benefit.

Interruptions to Infusions

Drotrecogin alfa (activated) should be stopped in the following situations:-

- Clinically significant bleeding – discuss with medical staff
- Procedures with a bleeding risk – discontinue drotrecogin alfa (activated) 2 hours prior to surgery or an invasive procedure (e.g. central venous lines, arterial lines, chest drains).
- Drotrecogin alfa (activated) may be restarted immediately after uncomplicated procedures and 12 hours after major invasive procedures if adequate haemostasis has been achieved. Remember that infusions made up more than 14 hours previously need to be discarded.

The infusion should run for a total of 96 hours. Any time missed due to interruptions should be accounted for during the infusion period.

Patients weighing less than 67 kg
Use a concentration of 100 microgram/ml (10 mg in 100 ml)

- Reconstitute each of 2 × 5 mg vials with 2.5 ml sterile water for injection (2 mg/ml)
- Gently swirl the vial – do not shake as this will cause frothing
- **Slowly** withdraw 5 ml from a 100 ml bag of sodium chloride 0.9% and discard
- **Slowly** add 5 ml of the reconstituted drotrecogin alfa (activated) to the infusion bag to give a final concentration of 10 mg in 100 ml (100 microgram/ml)
- Invert the bag **gently** to mix
- Infuse at 24 microgram/kg/hour at the appropriate rate below:

Patient Weight (kg)	Rate of Infusion (ml/hour)	Approximate time for 100 ml to be administered (hours)	Number of vials needed for 96 hours
40	9.6	10	19
45	10.8	9	21
50	12	8	24
55	13.2	8	26
60	14.4	7	28
65	15.6	6	30

Patients weight of 67 to 135 kg
Use a concentration of 200 microgram/ml (20 mg in 100 ml)

- Reconstitute each of 4×5 mg vials with 2.5 ml sterile water for injection (2 mg/ml)
- Gently swirl the vial – do not shake as this will cause frothing
- **Slowly** withdraw 10 ml from a 100 ml bag of 0.9% sodium chloride and discard
- **Slowly** add the reconstituted drotrecogin alfa (activated) to the infusion bag to give a final concentration of 20 mg in 100 ml (200 microgram/ml)
- Invert the bag **gently** to mix
- Infuse at 24 microgram/kg/hour at the appropriate rate below:

Patient Weight (kg)	Rate of Infusion (ml/hour)	Approximate time for 100 ml to be administered (hours)	Number of vials needed for 96 hours
70	8.4	12	36
75	9	11	36
80	9.6	10	40
85	10.2	10	40
90	10.8	9	44
95	11.4	9	44
100	12	8	48
110	13.2	8	52
120	14.4	7	56
130	15.6	6	60

APPENDIX J: DROTRECOGIN ADMINISTRATION RECORD

Intensive Care Unit   York Hospitals **NHS**

NHS Trust

Administration record for drotrecogin alfa (activated) (Xigris™)

| Patient name |
| Address |

Date of birth   Hospital no.

Patients weight .... kg

Date infusion started □ □ □ □   Time infusion started □ □ : □ □

Infusion duration (hours)	Tick when completed
1	
2	
3	
4	
5	
6	
7	
8	
9	
10	

Infusion duration (hours)	Tick when completed
25	
26	
27	
28	
29	
30	
31	
32	
33	
34	

Infusion duration (hours)	Tick when completed
49	
50	
51	
52	
53	
54	
55	
56	
57	
58	

Infusion duration (hours)	Tick when completed
73	
74	
75	
76	
77	
78	
79	
80	
81	
82	

(Continued)

11		
12		
13		
14		
15		
16		
17		
18		
19		
20		
21		
22		
23		
24		

35		
36		
37		
38		
39		
40		
41		
42		
43		
44		
45		
46		
47		
48		

59		
60		
61		
62		
63		
64		
65		
66		
67		
68		
69		
70		
71		
72		

83		
84		
85		
86		
87		
88		
89		
90		
91		
92		
93		
94		
95		
96		

Interruptions

1) Date infusion stopped   ☐☐ ☐☐ ☐☐☐☐   Time infusion stopped   ☐☐ : ☐☐

    Reason for interruption ....

    Date infusion restarted   ☐☐ ☐☐ ☐☐☐☐   Time infusion restarted   ☐☐ : ☐☐

    Duration of interruption (hours : mins)   ☐☐ : ☐☐

(Continued)

263

Interruptions (continued)

2) Date infusion stopped ☐☐ ☐☐ ☐☐☐☐   Time infusion stopped ☐☐ : ☐☐

Reason for interruption ....

Date infusion restarted ☐☐ ☐☐ ☐☐☐☐   Time infusion restarted ☐☐ : ☐☐

Duration of interruption (hours : mins) ☐☐ : ☐☐

3) Date infusion stopped ☐☐ ☐☐ ☐☐☐☐   Time infusion stopped ☐☐ : ☐☐

Reason for interruption ....

Date infusion restarted ☐☐ ☐☐ ☐☐☐☐   Time infusion restarted ☐☐ : ☐☐

Duration of interruption (hours : mins) ☐☐ : ☐☐

(Continued)

4) Date infusion stopped ☐☐ ☐☐ ☐☐☐☐   Time infusion stopped ☐☐ : ☐☐

Reason for interruption ....

Date infusion restarted ☐☐ ☐☐ ☐☐☐☐   Time infusion restarted ☐☐ : ☐☐

Duration of interruption (hours : mins) ☐☐ : ☐☐

5) Date infusion stopped ☐☐ ☐☐ ☐☐☐☐   Time infusion stopped ☐☐ : ☐☐

Reason for interruption ....

Date infusion restarted ☐☐ ☐☐ ☐☐☐☐   Time infusion restarted ☐☐ : ☐☐

Duration of interruption (hours : mins) ☐☐ : ☐☐

Senna - soften

Lactulose - ↑ H_2O in bowel.

DRUG INDEX

Proprietary (trade) names are printed in *italics*.

DRUG INDEX

DRUG INDEX

WH notes

APTR every 4/6 hours
   if on heparin.

if heparin amount
   changed, check every 1/2 hrs